Providing Healthy and Safe Foods As We Age

Workshop Summary

AF903863

Leslie Pray, Caitlin Boon, Emily Ann Miller, and
Laura Pillsbury, *Rapporteurs*

Food Forum

Food and Nutrition Board

INSTITUTE OF MEDICINE
OF THE NATIONAL ACADEMIES

THE NATIONAL ACADEMIES PRESS
Washington, D.C.
www.nap.edu

THE NATIONAL ACADEMIES PRESS 500 Fifth Street, N.W. Washington, DC 20001

NOTICE: The project that is the subject of this report was approved by the Governing Board of the National Research Council, whose members are drawn from the councils of the National Academy of Sciences, the National Academy of Engineering, and the Institute of Medicine.

This study was supported by Contract No. HHSF22301004T (U.S. Department of Health and Human Services and the Interagency Risk Assessment Consortium); AG-3A94-P-09-0172 and OEM-09-DC-01 (U.S. Department of Agriculture), N01-OD-4-2139 (National Institutes of Health), and HHSF22301005T (Food and Drug Administration) between the National Academy of Sciences. Additional support came from Abbott Laboratories, Campbell Soup, Cargill, Coca-Cola Company, ConAgra Foods, General Mills, Kellogg Company, Kraft Foods, Mars, McDonalds, Mead Johnson Nutrition, Monsanto, and PepsiCo. Any opinions, findings, conclusions, or recommendations expressed in this publication are those of the author(s) and do not necessarily reflect the view of the organizations or agencies that provided support for this project.

International Standard Book Number-13: 978-0-309-15883-1
International Standard Book Number-10: 0-309-15883-4

Additional copies of this report are available from the National Academies Press, 500 Fifth Street, N.W., Lockbox 285, Washington, DC 20055; (800) 624-6242 or (202) 334-3313 (in the Washington metropolitan area); Internet, http://www.nap.edu.

For more information about the Institute of Medicine, visit the IOM home page at **www.iom.edu.**

Printed in the United States of America

The serpent has been a symbol of long life, healing, and knowledge among almost all cultures and religions since the beginning of recorded history. The serpent adopted as a logotype by the Institute of Medicine is a relief carving from ancient Greece, now held by the Staatliche Museen in Berlin.

Suggested citation: IOM (Institute of Medicine). 2010. *Providing Healthy and Safe Foods as We Age: Workshop Summary.* Washington, DC: The National Academies Press.

"Knowing is not enough; we must apply.
Willing is not enough; we must do."
—Goethe

INSTITUTE OF MEDICINE
OF THE NATIONAL ACADEMIES

Advising the Nation. Improving Health.

THE NATIONAL ACADEMIES

Advisers to the Nation on Science, Engineering, and Medicine

The **National Academy of Sciences** is a private, nonprofit, self-perpetuating society of distinguished scholars engaged in scientific and engineering research, dedicated to the furtherance of science and technology and to their use for the general welfare. Upon the authority of the charter granted to it by the Congress in 1863, the Academy has a mandate that requires it to advise the federal government on scientific and technical matters. Dr. Ralph J. Cicerone is president of the National Academy of Sciences.

The **National Academy of Engineering** was established in 1964, under the charter of the National Academy of Sciences, as a parallel organization of outstanding engineers. It is autonomous in its administration and in the selection of its members, sharing with the National Academy of Sciences the responsibility for advising the federal government. The National Academy of Engineering also sponsors engineering programs aimed at meeting national needs, encourages education and research, and recognizes the superior achievements of engineers. Dr. Charles M. Vest is president of the National Academy of Engineering.

The **Institute of Medicine** was established in 1970 by the National Academy of Sciences to secure the services of eminent members of appropriate professions in the examination of policy matters pertaining to the health of the public. The Institute acts under the responsibility given to the National Academy of Sciences by its congressional charter to be an adviser to the federal government and, upon its own initiative, to identify issues of medical care, research, and education. Dr. Harvey V. Fineberg is president of the Institute of Medicine.

The **National Research Council** was organized by the National Academy of Sciences in 1916 to associate the broad community of science and technology with the Academy's purposes of furthering knowledge and advising the federal government. Functioning in accordance with general policies determined by the Academy, the Council has become the principal operating agency of both the National Academy of Sciences and the National Academy of Engineering in providing services to the government, the public, and the scientific and engineering communities. The Council is administered jointly by both Academies and the Institute of Medicine. Dr. Ralph J. Cicerone and Dr. Charles M. Vest are chair and vice chair, respectively, of the National Research Council.

www.national-academies.org

PLANNING COMMITTEE FOR FOOD SUPPLY AND AGING POPULATIONS[1]

SUSAN J. CROCKETT (*Co-chair*), General Mills, Minneapolis, MN
STEVE GENDEL (*Co-chair*), U.S. Food and Drug Administration, College Park, MD
KERRY DEARFIELD, U.S. Department of Agriculture, Washington, DC
GORDON L. JENSEN, Pennsylvania State University, University Park, PA
MARGARET LEAHY, The Coca-Cola Company, Atlanta, GA
PAMELA STARKE-REED, National Institutes of Health, Bethesda, MD

Study Staff

CAITLIN BOON, Study Director (through August 2010)
LAURA PILLSBURY, Study Director (from August 2010)
EMILY ANN MILLER, Research Associate
GERALDINE KENNEDO, Administrative Assistant
LINDA MEYERS, Director, Food and Nutrition Board

[1] Institute of Medicine planning committees are solely responsible for organizing the workshop, identifying topics, and choosing speakers. The responsibility for the published workshop summary rests with the workshop rapporteurs and the institution.

FOOD FORUM[1]

[1] Institute of Medicine forums and roundtables do not issue, review, or approve individual documents. The responsibility for the published workshop summary rests with the workshop rapporteurs and the institution.

Reviewers

This report has been reviewed in draft form by individuals chosen for their diverse perspectives and technical expertise, in accordance with procedures approved by the National Research Council's Report Review Committee. The purpose of this independent review is to provide candid and critical comments that will assist the institution in making its published report as sound as possible and to ensure that the report meets institutional standards for objectivity, evidence, and responsiveness to the study charge. The review comments and draft manuscript remain confidential to protect the integrity of the process. We wish to thank the following individuals for their review of this report:

Gordon L. Jensen, Department of Nutritional Sciences, Pennsylvania State University
Robert M. Russell, former Director, Jean Mayer Human Nutrition Research Center on Aging, Tufts University
Linda G. Snetselaar, Department of Preventive Medicine and Environmental Health, University of Iowa
Pamela Starke-Reed, Division of Nutrition Research Coordination, National Institutes of Health
Martin Wiedmann, Department of Food Science, Cornell University

Although the reviewers listed above have provided many constructive comments and suggestions, they did not endorse the final draft of the report before its release. The review of this report was overseen by **Melvin Worth.** Appointed by the Institute of Medicine, he was responsible for making certain that an independent examination of this report was carried out in accordance with institutional procedures and that all review comments were carefully considered. Responsibility for the final content of this report rests entirely with the authors and the institution.

Contents

Overview

With baby boomers reaching their 50s and 60s and the growth rate of the U.S. population age 65 years and older expected to double over the next twenty years, the need to prepare for an expanding population of older adults has never been as urgent as it is now. The growing size and changing demographics of aging adults place new demands on the food supply, with older adults not only being more susceptible to certain foodborne illnesses or health complications caused by those illnesses but also likely to experience significant changes in dietary needs and nutrition. While there is still a great deal to learn about what constitutes an "optimal diet" for older adults, available evidence indicates that dietary needs change with aging as a result of sensory loss and other physiological changes, changes in food preparation, and other eating-related behaviors. The fast-growing nature of the U.S. older population also creates new communication challenges with respect to educating older adults about how to manage a nutritious diet, how to prepare and store food safely, and how to act in the event of a safety-related food recall. In recognition of these trends and challenges, the Institute of Medicine's (IOM's) Food Forum convened a one-and-a-half-day workshop in October 2009 to explore food supply issues of relevance to aging adults. Specifically, the purpose of the workshop was to address the questions: What are the future challenges to providing healthy and safe foods to aging populations, and what can be done to meet those challenges?

Jointly sponsored by the Interagency Risk Assessment Consortium (IRAC),[1] the Food and Drug Administration's (FDA's) Center for Food Safety and Applied Nutrition (CFSAN), and the Food Forum, the workshop served as an opportunity for experts in various disciplines to discuss the size, demographics, and health status of community-dwelling populations more than 50 years of age; bring attention to the food safety and nutritional concerns that arise in these populations; and provide insight on how new food processing and reformulation technologies and consumer messaging can be used as preventive approaches to reducing the food and nutritional concerns for this growing segment of the U.S. population.

Food Forum Chair Michael Doyle opened the meeting with some brief introductory remarks about the general role of the IOM Food Forum and the objectives of the workshop. He also identified the planning committee responsible for organizing the workshop: Suzie J. Crockett of General Mills; Kerry Dearfield, U.S. Department of Agriculture (USDA), Food Safety and Inspection Service (FSIS); Steven Gendel, FDA/CFSAN; Gordon Jensen, Department of Nutritional Sciences, Pennsylvania State University; Marge Leahy, The Coca-Cola Company; and Pamela Starke-Reed, National Institutes of Health (NIH) Division of Nutrition Research Coordination (DNRC).

Doyle's comments were followed by an introductory presentation by Stephen Sundlof, Director of FDA/CFSAN. The remainder of the workshop was organized into six sessions: (1) size and demographics of aging populations; (2) changes in physiology with age; (3) food safety concerns for aging populations; (4) nutrition concerns for aging populations; (5) communicating with aging populations; and (6) future challenges and solutions to providing healthy and safe foods to aging populations. The final session included a panel discussion amongst four panelists and the audience. Many of the major themes of the workshop were revisited during this final session.

The organization of this report parallels the organization of the workshop itself. The introductory chapter, Chapter 1, includes a summary of Dr. Stephen Sundlof's presentation and a summary of the major overarching themes of the workshop presentations and discussions. Chapter 2 summarizes the presentations and the discussion that occurred during the session on size and demographics of aging populations (i.e., session 1), Chapter 3 summarizes the presentations and discussion of the session on changes in physiology with age (i.e., session 2), and so on. Summaries of the major themes of the workshop, including suggestions put forth by individual participants

---

[1] Founded in 1997, IRAC comprises all federal agencies, institutes, and centers with risk analysis responsibilities for food safety. Information about IRAC members and activities is available online at http://www.foodrisk.org/IRAC/.

for possible solutions to some of the key challenges to improving nutrition and food safety in older adults, can be found in Chapters 1 and 7.

The meeting transcripts and presentations served as basis for the summary. These proceedings summarize only the statements of workshop participants and are not intended to be an exhaustive exploration of the subject matter. The agenda for the workshop appears in Appendix A, and Appendix B lists the workshop participants. Appendix C contains the biographical sketches for the presenters, moderators, and panelists. Appendix D lists acronyms and abbreviations used throughout the workshop.

The reader should be aware that the materials presented here express the views and opinions of individuals participating in the workshop either as presenters, panelists, or audience members, and not the deliberations or conclusions of a formally constituted IOM committee. The objective of the workshop was not to come to consensus on any particular issue or formulate recommendations for future action. The goal was to illuminate issues, not resolve them. Nor was the objective to comprehensively address all food supply issues of relevance to aging adults, although the workshop did cover a very broad spectrum of some of the most important issues. Rather, the goal was to serve as a mechanism for individuals from a variety of government, academic, industry, and citizen groups to discuss and debate issues openly and identify possible approaches for addressing some of the most pressing food safety, nutrition, and communication issues of relevance to aging adults.

It should be noted at the outset that there were questions raised but no decision made about the most appropriate language to use when discussing aging populations. Different presenters used different terms, ranging from "mature" to "senior" to "elderly." Part of the language problem stems from the fact that aging is not something that begins at a certain age, rather it is a lifetime process, as several workshop participants emphasized. When asked when "old age" begins, people respond differently depending on their own age. When discussing an "aging population," some people may have in mind the population age 65 years and older, while others may be referring to the population age 50 and older and still others the population age 85 and older. Also, some workshop participants mentioned not wanting to use offensive language when referring to older adults, although there was no discussion around what would be considered offensive. One of the most commonly used terms was "older adult." While the rapporteurs of this workshop summary used many of these terms interchangeably, they likewise favored "older adult." This summary highlights the dramatic differences between older adults ages 50 to 65 and adults age 85 and above.

1

Introduction

While the goal of the workshop was neither to reach consensus on any single issue nor make specific recommendations about how to resolve any of these issues, several main themes emerged over the course of the one-and-a-half-day dialogue. This chapter provides an overview of the major themes of the workshop presentations as well as a summary of Stephen Sundlof's introductory presentation. The workshop presentations encompassed a wide range of themes from the current state-of-the-science on aging populations to potential opportunities and directions for the future. For one, America's aging population is actually many different aging populations (i.e., with respect to age but also socioeconomic status, level of family support, etc.). On the other hand, some presenters noted that although stakeholders across sectors are increasing their focus on food safety, nutrition, and food communication with older adults, there is both a need and opportunity for these different stakeholders to join forces and collaborate in ways that could accelerate progress. Sundlof's presentation focused largely on actions that the U.S. Food and Drug Administration (FDA) has already taken or is planning for the future with respect to improving not just food safety but also nutrition. Many of those actions revolve around nutrition labeling on packaged foods. Actions aimed at improving dietary choices among older adults in particular include conducting age-related risk assessments and developing educational materials and messages aimed at older adults.

MAIN THEMES OF WORKSHOP DISCUSSION

Again, while the goal of the workshop was neither to reach consensus on any single issue nor make specific recommendations about how to resolve any of these issues, several overarching themes emerged from the workshop presentations:

- *Government, private industry, and academia are all increasing their focus on food safety, nutrition, and communication in older adults.* In his overview, Sundlof described various FDA initiatives aimed at improving food safety and nutrition in older adults. Later, a wide range of other government, academic, and industry representatives discussed the variety of ways that different stakeholders are embracing the challenge of improving food safety and nutrition in aging populations.
- *America's aging population is actually many aging populations.* As Kevin Kinsella discussed during his presentation, there is tremendous heterogeneity in the U.S. population of adults more than 65 years old with respect not just to age (e.g., 65-and-over vs. 85-and-over) but to race, socioeconomic status, level of family support, disability, chronic health conditions, and other factors. This theme was revisited several times during the workshop and in several different contexts. For example, as discussed during the session on changes in physiology with age (see Chapter 3), the sensory and physiological changes that accompany aging and the implications of these changes with respect to both food safety and nutrition can be dramatically different between someone in his or her fifties versus someone who is 80 years of age or older. As people age, their susceptibility to certain foodborne illnesses changes, as does their overall nutritional status. As another example, discussed at length during the final session of the workshop (see Chapter 7), older adults have varying levels of family support. The majority of older adults live in the community, raising important questions about the strength (or, as one participant questioned, the existence) of the infrastructure in place for providing nutrition services to these adults. Simultaneously, the fact that a small but significant percentage of older adults live in assisted living facilities or other settings also raises equally important questions about the quality of nutritional services that this segment of the older population is receiving.
- *Aging is a lifetime process.* Related to the previous themes, there were several remarks about how aging begins during early development and not at any particular age later in life. For example, Luigi Fontana elaborated on this notion during his presentation on caloric

restriction. It was suggested that when discussions occur around aging, it should be clearly stated what particular age group is under consideration.

- *Aging is accompanied by a wide range of physiological changes, with varied implications for what can and should be done to improve food safety and nutrition in older adults.* For example, Simin Meydani elaborated on how the immune system changes with age, making older adults more susceptible to infectious disease and presented evidence from several studies suggesting that nutritional manipulation could decrease susceptibility to infection in older adults. Steven Gendel argued, on the other hand, that there is more to infection than an impaired immune system. He described evidence showing that not all foodborne pathogens are of concern and that susceptibility varies, with some microbes of greater concern than others. He emphasized that while monitoring for disease incidence can have a significant public health impact, it is important to recognize that there are two factors to consider when determining whether a foodborne pathogen poses a risk to older adults and that the two factors are not necessarily linked—(1) incidence and (2) severity of illness. Gordon Jensen discussed that while most of the gastrointestinal (GI) system remains largely intact as people age, with most serious dysfunction being related to an underlying health condition, the one component of GI function that does tend to degrade with aging is oral health (e.g., changes in dentition and swallowing). Not only does impaired oral health lead to poor diet quality and micronutrient deficiencies, periodontal disease in particular has been associated with an increased risk of cardiovascular disease. Finally, Marcia Pelchat described how three different sensory perceptions (taste, olfaction, and "chemical feeling") change with age and impact eating. For example, pleasant flavors becoming less pleasant and unpleasant flavors becoming less unpleasant, the latter leading to a loss of taste's gate-keeping function for protecting the body (e.g., the ability to detect food spoilage or salt).
- *While industry has made tremendous progress in developing new food processing techniques and novel packaging that minimize many food safety problems, there are still important unanswered questions about how food processing, formulation, and packaging can be improved to better meet the needs of older adults.* Michael Doyle discussed some of the innovative food processing technologies that have been designed to protect food and minimize contamination and other food safety problems, as well as some of the challenges that still exist. Aaron Brody described the wide range of packaging technologies designed to do the same. Brody's talk in particular

prompted several questions about some of the challenges that still exist with respect to developing innovative packaging that works well for older consumers.

- *While most of the workshop participants who commented on the issue agreed that high quality diets and nutrient optimization are necessary for maintaining good health in older adults, several questions remain about exactly what constitutes a high quality diet (e.g., should older adults eat more or less protein?) and obstacles to obtaining that optimal diet (e.g., poor oral health, loss of appetite).* Katherine Tucker discussed how dietary needs change with age and identified some of the challenges with meeting those needs; Stephen Barnes discussed functional foods (i.e., foods that promote health) and bioavailability challenges for older adults; and Luigi Fontana discussed the role of caloric restriction in regulating many biological factors known to be associated with aging.
- *There are many unanswered research questions and a lack of data around food safety and nutrition concerns in older adults.* Lack of data is a serious problem not just with respect to gaining a better understanding of the nutritional needs of older adults but for many other issues as well. For example, in the final session of the workshop (see Chapter 7), Steven Gendel remarked that one of the challenges with differentiating among multiple aging populations is the lack of health monitoring data and the consequent inability to generate enough statistical power to make conclusions about the health conditions and needs of those varied populations. As another example, Bernadene Magnuson presented recent findings on the adverse effects of soy and curcumin and argued that many active ingredients in dietary supplements are understudied and may have unknown safety risks. David Greenblatt, on the other hand, in his telling of "the grapefruit story" (how grapefruit juice interacts with some drugs), argued that ample data on CYP3A (the enzyme responsible for the grapefruit juice-drug interaction) implicate only very few interactions between food in general and drugs.
- *Communication is an important component of improving nutrition in older adults, with many ongoing industry-sponsored programs aimed at elucidating the best way to communicate about nutrition to older adults.* For example, Steven Bodhaine described what a recent wellness segmentation study revealed about how older adults view health and food, emphasizing the need to engage consumers on a personal level. Jim Kirkwood described the results of studies that General Mills has conducted in an effort to learn what drives consumers' food choices, emphasizing the importance of combining scientific facts about nutrition with "the things that really matter

to consumers" when developing and marketing new food products. More generally, Ronni Chernoff listed and described the key elements of effective written and oral communication.

- Similarly, *communication is an important component of improving food safety in older adults, and there are many unanswered questions around how to best communicate about food safety issues with older adults.* William Hallman discussed lessons learned from recent surveys on how people respond to food recalls and emphasized the need to "get it right," given that food recalls are likely to become even more frequent in the future as the food supply continues to expand (globally) and food surveillance technologies continue to advance. Caroline Smith DeWaal emphasized the potential value of on-the-spot messaging when communicating urgent food safety messages to older adults, as well as the value of restaurant grading systems. Both talks prompted several questions about the need to devise new means of risk communication when a recall or other urgent food safety event arises.
- *Most older adults live in the community, not in nursing homes or other institutional settings, and there is some concern that the infrastructure currently in place is insufficient for meeting the food safety and nutrition needs of this population.* Nancy Wellman elaborated on this reality and its implications during her presentation. The theme was revisited at length in the final panel session. At the same time, a smaller but significant proportion of the aging population, particularly the 85-and-over population, live in assisted living or other institutional settings, and some participants expressed concern about the quality of nutritional services that they are receiving.
- *There is enormous opportunity for collaboration between the food and food packaging industries and other food safety and nutrition stakeholders (academia, government, consumer groups) in efforts to address some of the most pressing food safety and nutrition issues in aging populations.* Suzie Crockett and several other participants touched on this theme throughout the workshop, citing examples of the ways that the U.S. government, industry, and the traditionally separate food safety and nutrition communities are already working together or could be working together to develop food products that meet the changing nutritional needs of older adults, devise new ways to communicate about food safety and nutrition to older adults, and tackle other pressing food safety and nutrition issues.

See Chapter 7 for a more detailed summary of some of these and other topics that were highlighted in the final session of the workshop, when four distinguished panelists were asked to comment on what they considered to be the most important issues and future challenges to providing healthy and safe foods to aging populations.

OVERVIEW OF THE CHALLENGES TO ENSURING SAFE AND NUTRITIOUS FOODS FOR AGING POPULATIONS

Presenter: Stephen Sundlof

Stephen Sundlof of the Center for Food Safety and Applied Nutrition (CFSAN) at FDA began by remarking on the necessity of accounting for aging populations when considering food safety. As such, FDA is increasingly taking aging into account when deliberating on food safety issues. FDA is also intensifying its focus on nutrition and has initiated or is planning many actions aimed at helping Americans of all ages make better dietary choices. The remainder of Sundlof's presentation focused on FDA's activity around nutrition.

First, he listed some pertinent facts about the current state of nutrition in the United States:

- Two-thirds of Americans are overweight or obese. Recent data indicate older adults, ages 50 to 69, are even more affected (Ogden et al., 2006; CDC, 2010).
- Diet and lifestyle choices are major causes of morbidity and mortality in the United States (especially from diabetes and heart disease).
- Most Americans do not meet the *Dietary Guidelines for Americans* recommendations with respect to their intake of fresh fruits and vegetables, which is known to be associated with lowering the risk for diabetes, heart disease, and other chronic diseases.
- Ninety percent of middle-aged Americans will develop high blood pressure at some point in their life, putting them at risk for hypertension, which can be controlled to some extent through diet.

Most of FDA's activity around nutrition involves the following:

- Reviewing and authorizing health claims and nutrient claims on labels so that consumers can make informed choices. FDA monitors about a dozen health claims, which must have sufficient scientific information in order to be considered as such (e.g., soluble fiber lowers cholesterol). The agency also monitors nutrient content claims, which must meet established criteria in order to be identified as such.

- Educating consumers about which foods comprise a healthful diet and which foods to moderate.
- Overseeing the labeling on packaged foods so that the information is neither false nor misleading.

Sundlof focused on the last activity: overseeing the labeling on packaged foods.

FDA Activity Around Nutrition: Overseeing Labeling on Packaged Foods

Sundlof identified the Nutrition Labeling and Education Act of 1990 (NLEA) as one of the most important recent milestones in FDA efforts to improve nutrition. NLEA makes the Nutrition Facts panel mandatory on the packaging of almost all foods, with the exception of individual snacks, fresh produce, and some other products. The panel contains nutrition information that helps consumers make informed choices about the healthfulness of their diets and usually is located on either the side or back of the package (see Figure 1-1). FDA is currently in the process of modernizing the panels

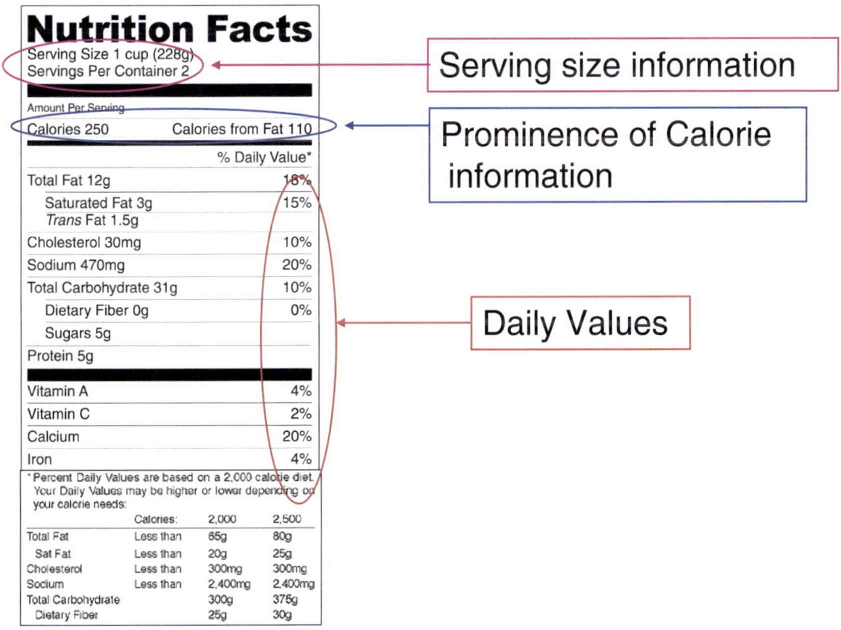

FIGURE 1-1 An example of a mandatory Nutrition Facts panel, with parts of the panel currently under review by FDA highlighted, as described by Sundlof.

based on public response. The agency recently issued an advance notice of proposed rulemaking, asking for comments on the panel and where improvements could be made (FDA/HHS, 2007). So far, among other lessons, FDA has learned

- *Serving size information* is often confusing, with serving sizes not equal to what people normally eat (e.g., a serving size of tortilla chips might be six chips, but few people sit down and eat only six chips). Many people do not even read the information. Serving size information needs to be improved such that the listed serving size is actually the same as what people normally consume in one sitting, and consumers need to be educated about what serving size means.
- Most people look at *calorie information* when seeking nutrition information, therefore FDA is working on ways to make this information more prominent. The agency is also considering eliminating "Calories from Fat" and replacing it with "Percent of Daily Value" information.
- *Daily Values* are due for reconsideration to see if they are still accurate, with some changes expected based on new information.

Point-of-Purchase Labeling

Given recent publicity around point-of-purchase labeling, which includes both front-of-package labeling and shelf labeling, Sundlof spoke in detail about measures FDA is implementing in an effort to manage confusing labeling. Food companies are increasingly including nutrition information not just in the Nutrition Facts panel but also on the front of packages given that this information can influence people's choices about which foods to buy. However, from what FDA has heard from the food industry, retailers, food processors, and others, the information becomes very confusing very quickly.

Front-of-package labels. There are two main types of front-of-package labels used in the United States:

- *Summary symbols*, which contain minimal information indicating that the food meets some kind of health criterion (e.g., it is "healthy" or "good for you"). Usually, the product is compared to other products within a product group. For example, many cereals contain symbols indicating that that they are "a better choice" than other cereals. There are a number of different types of front-of-package symbols being used. For example, the "Smart Choices" label, developed by a consortium of private, public health, and academic nutrition leaders, has received much attention recently.[1] Just a couple weeks prior to the workshop, the Smart Choices program announced that it would no longer be accepting additional clients. Sundlof explained that, according to a public statement by the U.S. Commissioner of Food and Drugs, Margaret Hamburg, FDA is not fully supportive of the criteria of the Smart Choices program. For example, some cereals have qualified even though their composition is nearly 50 percent sugar. Sundlof said that following Hamburg's statement, many major food companies announced they would no longer be participating in the Smart Choices program. Also, just prior to the workshop, Hamburg indicated FDA would be looking into developing a single front-of-package system in an effort to minimize the confusion associated with the wide range of labeling systems currently in use.

- *Nutrient specific symbols*, whereby the front of the package provides information about specific nutrients (e.g., fiber, sugar, calories).

Sundlof pointed to the United Kingdom Food Standards Agency's voluntary traffic light system as an example of a different type of front-of-package labeling: symbols that provide both specific nutrition information and gradations about positive or negative levels of fat, saturated fat, salt, and sugars.[2] A red light indicates a high level, an amber light a medium level, and green light a low level. Traffic light symbols provide consumers with a lot of information that can be gathered in a glance. Because it is a voluntary system, it tends not to be used for products that would have a lot of red lights. However, because the United Kingdom does not require nutrition fact labeling, this is one of the few ways that consumers can view information about the nutrition content of foods. The system has garnered some attention in the United States and is being considered as a possible option according to Sundlof.

Shelf labeling. Sundlof mentioned the "Guiding Stars" system, developed by Hannaford Supermarkets, as example of shelf labeling: the more stars, the "healthier" the food under Guiding Stars criteria.[3]

---

[1] More information about the Smart Choices program, including its nutrition criteria, is available online at http://www.smartchoicesprogram.com/.

[2] More information about traffic light labeling in the United Kingdom can be found online at http://www.eatwell.gov.uk/foodlabels/trafficlights/.

[3] More information on the Guiding Stars shelf-tag labeling system is available online at http://www.guidingstars.com/.

FDA Actions

In an effort to alleviate some of the confusion around point-of-purchase labeling, FDA is

- analyzing front-of-package labels that appear to be misleading and determining what type of regulatory action needs to be taken to prevent consumers from being misled;
- reviewing nutrient-specific front-of-package labels to ensure that they are consistent with the regulatory criteria established for the nutrient content claim (e.g., if the label indicates that the food is low fat, the food must be low in fat as defined by FDA);
- developing a proposed rule to standardize front-of-package labeling and provide consistent criteria for use of the labeling (i.e., whether or not a single front-of-package label is developed, the criteria should nonetheless be consistent); and
- conducting research on how consumers view and use front-of-package labeling and whether individuals make good diet choices based on labeling (e.g., while consumers are more likely to purchase a product with front-of-package labeling, versus a product without such labeling, it is unclear whether this behavior actually contributes to building a healthier diet).

FDA FOOD SAFETY AND NUTRITION ACTIONS AIMED SPECIFICALLY AT AGING POPULATIONS

FDA is implementing several measures aimed specifically at improving dietary choices among older adults, including the following:

- Considering age-related issues when conducting safety and risk assessments. For example, when examining a new food additive or responding to the detection of a contaminant, the agency considers not just the general population but also subpopulations and then makes decisions based on the most sensitive subpopulation(s).
- Monitoring adverse event data for problems affecting specific age groups.
- Developing educational materials and safety messages aimed at seniors and their caregivers. For example, www.foodsafety.gov (a new website developed by the White House Food Safety Working Group and which contains both U.S. Department of Agriculture [USDA] and FDA food safety information) and www.fda.gov provide consumer publications and other information on food safety and nutrition for seniors. For example, among other information FDA's "Resources for You: Food

> Safety for Seniors" webpage[4] provides senior consumers with a list of foods to avoid: raw fin fish and shellfish (because of the many infectious agents that they can transmit), hot dogs and luncheon meats unless reheated until steaming hot (because of *Listeria*), raw or unpasteurized milk or soft cheeses (because of *Listeria*), refrigerated pates or meat spreads (again, because of *Listeria*), raw or lightly cooked eggs or egg products (because of *Salmonella*), raw meat or poultry (because of *Salmonella)*, raw sprouts (because of *Salmonella*, *Listeria,* and *E. Coli*), and unpasteurized or untreated fruit or vegetable juice (because of *E. coli* O157:H7). FDA has also issued a publication, "Using the Nutrition Facts Label: A How-To Guide for Older Adults," and is developing Fight BAC![5] materials aimed at different age groups.

In conclusion, Sundlof emphasized that FDA is strengthening its focus on nutrition, especially among older adults, and is making a major effort toward improving nutrition labeling so that consumers of all ages can make healthier dietary choices. He stressed that success will depend on a team effort and partnerships between FDA and other agencies and organizations.

QUESTIONS AND DISCUSSION

Sundlof's presentation prompted several questions about how FDA gathers its consumer information (i.e., with respect to what consumers would like to see on nutrition panels); whether FDA foresees developing a different type of food nutrition labeling for older adults (e.g., with larger font sizes); and how decisions are made about some of the information that is included, or not included, on food labels (e.g., the lack of differentiation among different types of sugars).

How FDA Gathers Consumer Information

Sundlof explained that in addition to having sent notices through the Federal Register requesting input on what changes consumers would like to see on the Nutrition Facts panel and nutrition labels, FDA will also be conducting focus groups and other types of consumer research. He emphasized that FDA cannot impose new rules without consumer research, as the agency bases all of its regulations on science.

---

[4] Available online: http://www.fda.gov/Food/ResourcesForYou/Consumers/Seniors/ucm182679.htm (accessed August 3, 2010).

[5] The Fight BAC! campaign is a food safety initiative designed to educate consumers about the four simple practices—clean, separate, cook, and chill—that can help reduce their risk of foodborne illness. The campaign was created by the Partnership for Food Safety Education (PFSE), and Fight BAC! materials can be accessed through www.foodsafety.gov.

Different Nutrition Labeling for Older Adults?

With respect to whether or not FDA foresees having different types of labels for older adults, Sundlof explained that the Agency's objective is to make sure that the information on the label is understood by all groups.

How FDA Makes Decisions About Nutrition Label Information

An audience member asked Sundlof whether FDA will be revisiting rounding errors and content claims that declare a product is low fat or zero fat even though it may have, for example, 0.4 grams (g) of fat per serving. Sundlof explained that, generally, even if the level of a nutrient is a fraction of a point below a certain predetermined level, a claim (e.g., "zero fat") could be made. However, FDA is currently revisiting some of those claims, in particular *trans* fat levels. Currently, if a product contains less than 0.5 g *trans* fat per 100 g food, a claim can be made that the product has zero *trans* fat. As the methodology for *trans* fat detection has improved since that rule was established, FDA is reconsidering how *trans* fat free claims are regulated.

Another member of the audience asked about some of the other ingredients, such as high fructose corn syrup, that are not currently included on the Nutrition Facts panel and whether FDA is considering including information about any additional nutrients. Sundlof said that, with respect to sugars, those sorts of distinctions are not made on the Nutrition Facts panel. However, ingredients like high fructose corn syrup do appear on the ingredient list. Additionally, depending on how current development of a new front-of-package labeling system proceeds, that type of information may in the future be included elsewhere on the package as well.

When asked about whether smaller processors might be exempt from any new front-of-package labeling requirements, Sundlof said that, generally, FDA makes exceptions for the Nutrition Facts panel based on certain criteria (e.g., if the product is being sold as an individual snack) and that this will likely be the case for front-of-package labeling.

Finally, there was a question about the legibility and size of the information provided on labels and whether FDA is considering if it is appropriate for aging populations. The questioner remarked, "The best information that is on the label is not usable if it is not legible." Sundlof explained how FDA currently requires that certain Nutrition Facts panel criteria be met, for example certain information must meet a minimum font size, and FDA will be testing various font sizes and other properties of front-of-package labeling to ensure that different age groups, both older and younger populations, can read the information. He said that one of the challenges with front-of-package labeling, particularly on small packages, is that the package front is "prime real estate."

2

Size and Demographics of Aging Populations

Following opening remarks by moderator Pamela Starke-Reed of the National Institutes of Health (NIH) Division of Nutrition Research Coordination, Bethesda, Maryland, two speakers addressed the changing size and demographics of the nation's aging populations. First, Kevin Kinsella of the National Institute on Aging (NIA), Bethesda, Maryland, described the tremendous heterogeneity in U.S. aging populations and identified key health and socioeconomic trends among these populations (e.g., less institutionalization than in the past and existence of sensory impairment concerns about oral health). Then, Nancy Wellman of the Friedman School of Nutrition Science and Policy, Tufts University, Boston, Massachusetts, discussed food shopping, preparation, and consumption habits of older adults, as well as food insecurity trends among older adults. She emphasized that most Americans age 65 years and older live not in nursing homes or other institutional settings but in the community and that most food and nutrition programs aimed at providing services for these community-dwelling older adults are under-funded or disregarded. The presentations provided a wealth of background information on aging populations and served as a point of reference for the remainder of the workshop presentations and discussions. Both Kinsella's observations about the heterogeneity among aging populations and Wellman's remarks about the need to provide better food and nutrition services to community-dwelling older adults resurfaced many times during later discussions.

OUR AGING POPULATION

Presenter: Kevin Kinsella

Kinsella remarked that he would be describing growth in what he called the "older population" (i.e., people age 65 years and older), not just in terms of numbers but also with respect to socioeconomic trends, which he noted as relevant when thinking about food safety and other food concerns.

Growth of the Older Population

Today, there are about 39.5 million people in the United States over the age of 65, including 5.6 million people over 85. While these numbers appear high, if they are considered in a historical context, starting in 1910 up until 2050 (using projected numbers for the population size from the present year until 2050), it is very clear that the current growth rate of both the 65-and-older and 85-and-older is in fact lower than it has ever been in the past century (Figure 2-1). But this is about to change. In the

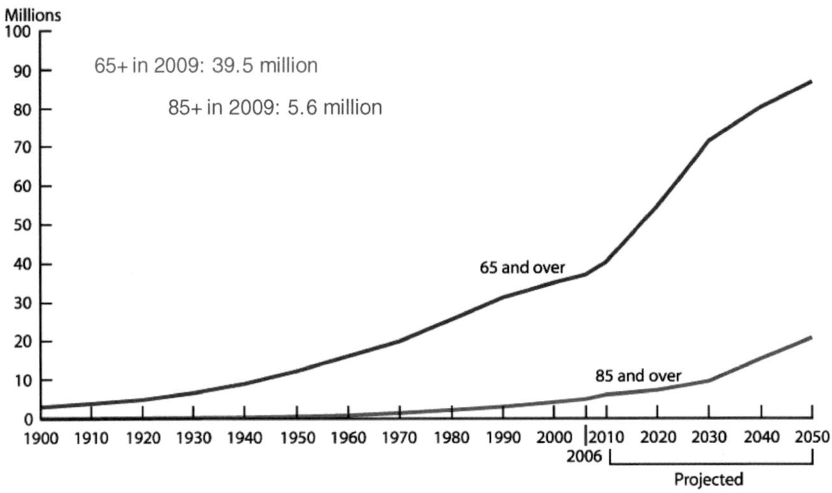

FIGURE 2-1 The U.S. populations, over time, of people more than 65 and 85 years of age.
NOTE: These data refer to the resident population; data for years 2010–2050 are projections of the population.
SOURCE: U.S. Census Bureau, Decennial Census, Population Estimates and Projections, 2008.

next one or two years and continuing over the course of the next 20 years, the growth rate of the older population is going to dramatically increase to nearly double what it is today (Figure 2-2). This steep incline reflects aging of the baby boomer generation, with about 75 million people moving into the ranks of the older population during the next 20 years.

Kinsella noted that the projected future growth of the 85-and-older population in particular has taken demographers and social scientists by surprise. By 2050, there will be an estimated 19 million people in the United States age 85 and older. In the past, statisticians have tended to underestimate improvements in mortality. If one were to examine these same projected numbers 20 years ago, the numbers would be a lot lower than they are today. But with improvements in mortality that have taken place over the past 40 or so years, by all accounts it appears that in fact this "oldest old" population (i.e., people age 85 and older) will grow tremendously over the next few decades. Moreover, given that these projected numbers are official U.S. Census Bureau numbers, Kinsella suspects that they may be conservative and that the real numbers could be even higher. Referring to discussion in the previous session about the legibility of food labels, Kinsella observed that this is an important trend to keep in mind, given the high prevalence of vision problems in the oldest old.

Kinsella discussed some key trends in the aging population in more detail. For example, geographically, the 65-and-older population is concentrated in the upper Midwest and parts of Florida. The 85-and-older population is concentrated in the upper Midwest, Florida, and New England. When categorized by race, from 2006 and projected to 2050, the

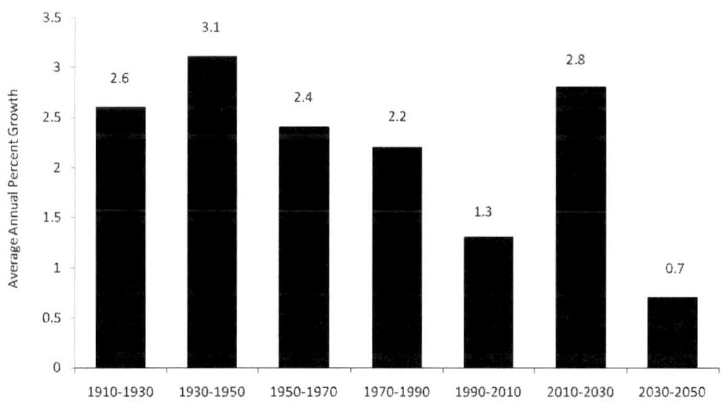

FIGURE 2-2 The changing growth rate of the U.S. population age 65 years and older.
SOURCE: U.S. Census Bureau, 2003.

non-Hispanic white population will become a much smaller percent of the total in the future (61 percent in 2050) than it is today (81 percent in 2006). Conversely, the Hispanic population will occupy a much larger proportion of the 65-and-older age group in the future (18 percent in 2050) than it does today (6 percent in 2006).

Kinsella explained how immigration is likely to impact the age structure of the U.S. population. Compared to other developed countries, the United States is a fairly young country in the sense that the proportion of the U.S. population that is 65 and older is fairly low and will remain fairly low in the future. The United States does not even rank among the top 20 countries with respect to the percentage of the population age 65 years or older because, although fertility rates in the United States tend to be slightly higher than in other developed countries, so do immigration rates. Every year, there is an influx of mostly young and middle-aged adults, with the bulk of the foreign-born U.S. population between the ages of 25 and 45 (Figure 2-3).

Just as life expectancy at birth has been increasing over the past century, so too has life expectancy at the ages of 65 and 85 (Figure 2-4). Kinsella explained that another way to examine this trend is to consider survivorship. Survival at every age has increased over the past century as well (Figure 2-5). In 1901, there was a large drop-off early in life because of infant mortality. Many people (up to about 20 percent) died during the

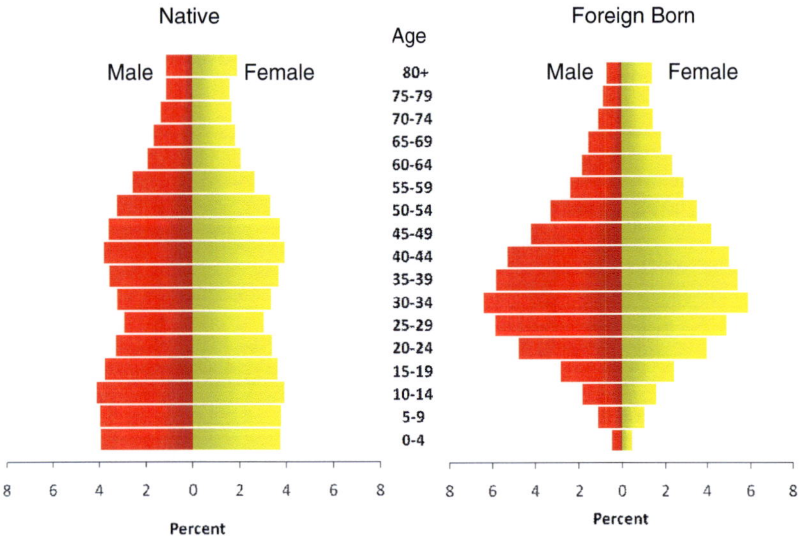

FIGURE 2-3 Age structure for the U.S. native- and foreign-born populations.
SOURCE: U.S. Current Population Survey, Annual Social and Economic Supplement, 2002.

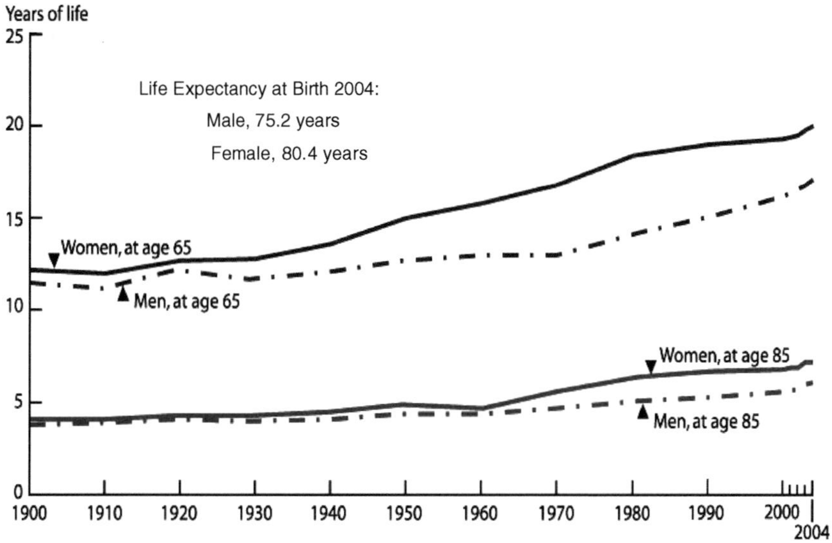

FIGURE 2-4 Life expectancy at ages 65 and 85 years, by sex, from the years 1900–2004.
NOTE: These data refer to the resident population.
SOURCE: National Vital Statistics System, 2008.

first one or two years of life. By 2004, this early drop-off all but disappeared. Meanwhile, survival at later ages has increased. For example, only 50 percent of white females survived to the age of 60 years in 1901, and only about 5 percent of white females who reached the age of 50 survived to the age of 90. In 2004, about 90 percent of white females survived to the age of 60, and more than 25 percent of white females who survived to the age of 50 survived to the age of 90.

Kinsella explained how the shift of the entire survivorship curve in Figure 2-5 has led to an interesting debate in gerontology with regard to what the future shape of the curve will look like. There is no sign that the trend is going to stop, but how far will it go? Will people be living to the age of 120 or 150? What are the limits to life expectancy?

Trends in Health in the Older Population

Kinsella raised the question: While it is clear the people are living longer, are they living any better? Are these added years healthy years, or does it mean that society will be experiencing more disease and disability? Until very recently, very few countries had data that could be used to de-

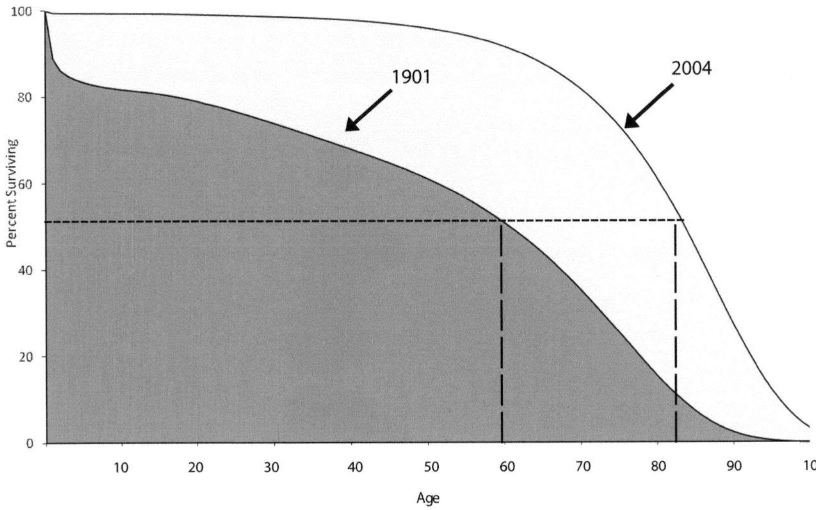

FIGURE 2-5 Survivorship curve among U.S. white females, for the years 1901 and 2004.
SOURCES: U.S. Census Bureau, 1936; National Center for Health Statistics (NCHS), 2007.

finitively answer these questions. Data from the U.S. National Longer-Term Care Surveys (NLTCS)[1] have only recently begun to provide some insight into disease and disability patterns and changes with aging. The good news, Kinsella said, is that non-disabled component of the Medicare-enrolled 65-and-over population has been rising over time. In 1982, 74 percent of Medicare-enrolled 65-and-older individuals were "non-disabled." That number rose to 81 percent in 2004–2005. This trend is reflected in the fact that the percentage of Medicare-enrolled 65-and-older individuals who reside in institutional settings (i.e., nursing homes) has decreased over time, to less than 5 percent in 2004–2005.

While largely non-disabled, substantial proportions of the older population nonetheless reported chronic conditions in the National Health Interview Survey. About half of all men (52 percent) and women (54 percent) over the age of 65 report hypertension (this does not include individuals with undiagnosed hypertension); and about half (43 percent of men, 54 percent

[1] NLTCS are nationally representative surveys of Medicare beneficiaries aged 65 and over with chronic functional disabilities. The first NLTCS survey was administered in 1982, with follow-up surveys conducted in 1984, 1989, 1994, 1999, and 2004. For more information, see http://www.nltcs.aas.duke.edu/ and http://aspe.hhs.gov/daltcp/reports/nltcssu2.htm.

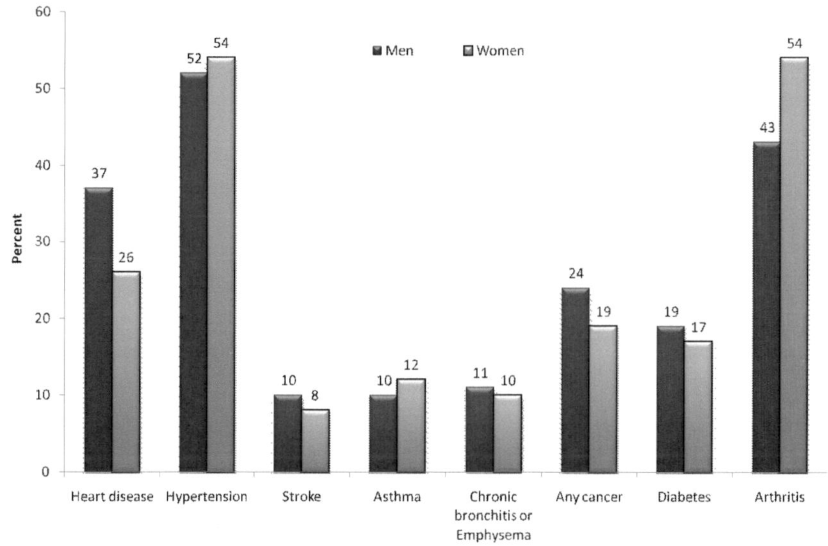

FIGURE 2-6 Percent of people age 65 and over who reported having selected chronic conditions, by sex, 2005–2006.
NOTE: Data are based on a 2-year average from 2005–2006 and refer to the civilian, non-institutionalized population.
SOURCE: NCHS, 2008.

of women) report arthritis (Figure 2-6). Overweight (defined as a body mass index [BMI] of 25 or greater) and obesity (BMI of 30 or greater) are also prevalent among the older population, with nearly 80 percent of men and 70 percent of women between the ages of 65 and 74 considered overweight according to the 2005–2006 National Health and Nutrition Examination Survey (NHANES).[2] Even in the 75-and-older populations, the levels of overweight are nearly as high. Importantly, the percentage of older adults who are overweight or obese has been increasing. Kinsella said obesity is not just a problem with "young kids eating a lot of junk food."

Many older adults also report problems with hearing, seeing, and oral health (Figure 2-7). Kinsella noted the high percentage of people over the age of 65 who have no natural teeth (about a quarter of the population), which he said is important to keep in mind when considering food consumption in the older population. Finally, a substantial proportion of the older population experiences at least some level of memory impairment, which may be important to keep in mind when considering how older adults decipher food messages and plan nutritional intake.

[2] Available online: http://www.cdc.gov/nchs/nhanes.htm (accessed August 23, 2010).

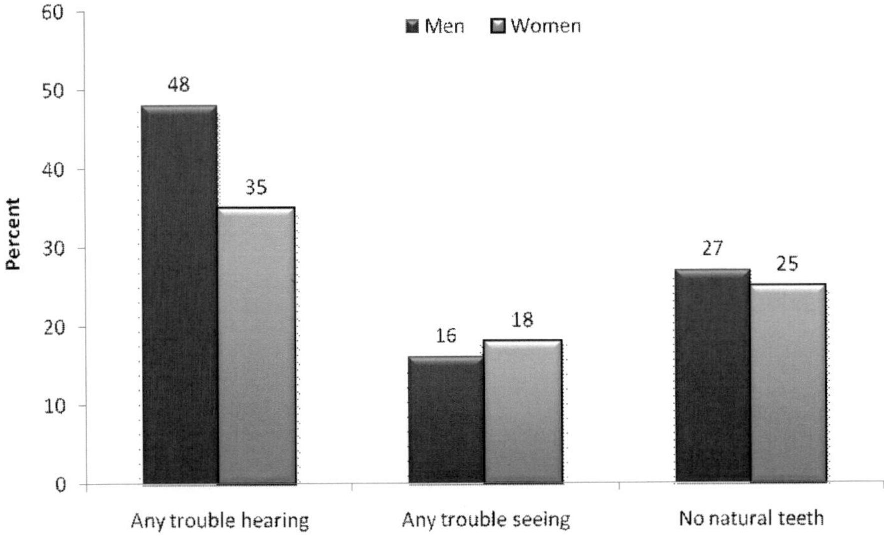

FIGURE 2-7 Percentage of people age 65 and older who reported having any trouble hearing, any trouble seeing, or no natural teeth, by sex, 2006.
NOTE: Respondents were asked "Which statement best describes your hearing without a hearing aid: good, a little trouble, a lot of trouble, deaf?" For the purposes of this indicator the category "Any trouble hearing" includes "a little trouble, a lot of trouble, and deaf." Regarding their vision, respondents were asked "Do you have any trouble seeing, even when wearing glasses or contact lenses?" The category "Any trouble seeing" also includes those who in a subsequent question report themselves as blind. Lastly, respondents were asked, in one question, "Have you lost all of your upper and lower natural (permanent) teeth?" Data refer to the civilian non-institutionalized population.
SOURCE: NCHS, 2008.

Socioeconomic Trends in the Older Population

Kinsella pointed out several socioeconomic indicators that may have some relevance to the workshop discussion:

- *Educational attainment.* In 1965, only about one quarter of individuals over the age of 65 had completed high school. Today, more than three-quarters of the older population has completed high school, with a much slower but noticeable increase in the percentage of older people who have attained bachelor's degrees as well.
- *Marital status.* While the current 65-and-older population has a relatively low percentage of people who are divorced or separated (around 9 percent), those figures are much higher for the 45–54 and 55–64 age

groups (around 18–19 percent). This means that, in the future, a much higher proportion of the older population will be divorced or separated, which will have implications for caregiving and social support.

- *Living alone*. A high percentage of older adults, particularly women (nearly 40 percent), live alone, which may have implications for food delivery, etc.
- *Poverty*. In the early 1960s, the older population had a higher proportion of people living in poverty than any other age group. Today, the older population has a lower proportion of people living in poverty than any other age group. Kinsella noted that Medicare, which was introduced in the early 1960s, seems to have had a rather important effect on alleviating poverty among older adults. He remarked that most of the poverty that does exist in the 65-and-older population is concentrated in the South and parts of the upper Midwest.
- *Food expenditure*. According to a 2005 survey by the Federal Forum on Aging Related Statistics,[3] people in all older age groups (55–64, 65–74, and 75-and-over) spend 13 percent of their total household annual expenditures on food.
- *Dietary quality*. According to a 2001–2002 survey by the same forum, Healthy Eating Index[4] scores are roughly the same for all older age groups (a score of 64 for 55-64 year olds and scores of 68 for the 65–74 and 75-and-over groups).

Lessons from Other Countries

In conclusion, Kinsella remarked on the value of looking at what other countries are doing to accommodate older populations. With the exception of Japan, which ranks as the world's oldest country (i.e., 21.6 percent of Japan's population is 65 years or older, which is higher than any other country), all of the other 25 oldest countries are in Europe (Figure 2-8). The United States is not even on the list. He pointed to the United Kingdom's traffic light labeling system for ranking ingredients in food products, which had been described in the introductory presentation by Steve Sundlof (see Chapter 1), as something that another country has successfully implemented in an effort to accommodate its growing older population and which may be something for the United States to consider. Kinsella suggested that there are probably other interesting and relevant

[3] Available online: www.agingstats.gov (accessed August 27, 2010).

[4] The Healthy Eating Index is a measure of diet quality that assesses conformity to U.S. federal dietary guidance. The components of the index and scoring standards are available online at: http://www.cnpp.usda.gov/Publications/HEI/healthyeatingindex2005factsheet.pdf.

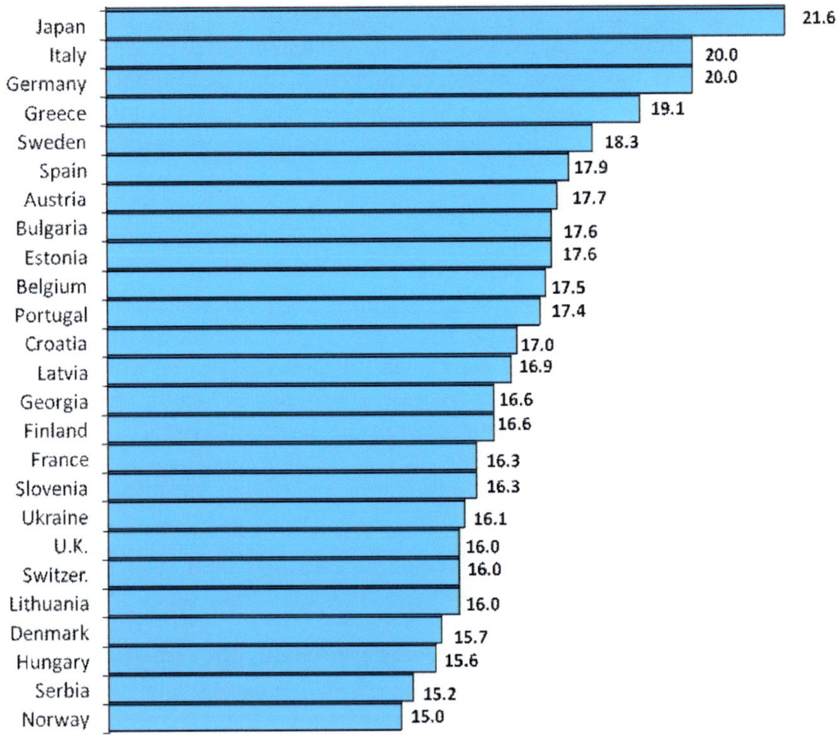

FIGURE 2-8 The world's 25 countries with the highest percentage of the population age 65 years or older.
SOURCE: U.S. Census Bureau, International Database, 2008.

initiatives under way in the countries in Figure 2-8 that we may benefit from knowing about.

FOOD PREPARATION AND CONSUMPTION HABITS OF COMMUNITY-DWELLING POPULATIONS

Presenter: Nancy Wellman

Wellman began her presentation by commenting on the fact that most Americans over the age of 65 live in the community, not in nursing homes or other institutions. Only 4.5 percent (about 1.5 million) of older adults live in nursing homes and 2 percent (1 million) in assisted living facilities. The majority of older adults (93.5 percent, or 33.4 million) live in the community. In fact, she remarked that it is U.S. federal policy to keep people out of nursing homes and to move people who currently live in nursing homes out of nursing homes, partly for budgetary reasons.[5] For the remainder of her presentation, she focused on food shopping, preparation, and consumption habits of older adults; food insecurity among older adults; and home and community-based food and nutrition programs that service older adults.

Food Shopping Behavior

First, Wellman shared data on various food shopping behaviors among all consumers (not differentiated by age) and among consumers age 55 years and older:

- *How much time shoppers (not differentiated by age) spend in different types of stores (grocery stores, dollar stores, etc.).* The time spent in stores varies, depending on the type of store and other variables such as frequency of shopping. For example, 36 percent of grocery store shopping trips last 15–30 minutes, but only 5 percent of convenience store shopping trips last that long.
- *How much time shoppers (not differentiated by age) spend in front of shelves looking at different foods.* Again, this varies, depending on food category and other variables such as whether the consumer has seen an advertisement for a product or is trying a new product. The average is around seven seconds, which Wellman described as "quick" and impinging on front-of-package and shelf labeling.
- *How shoppers 55 years and older use information on food packaging labels to make decisions.* Based on surveys conducted by the International Food Information Council Foundation (IFIC),[6] older adults generally tend to look at the Nutrition Facts panel, the expiration date, and the ingredient list and are not as concerned with other features such as brand name, country of origin, and whether a product is organic. Figure 2-9 illustrates these concerns.
- *What type of information shoppers 55 years and older are looking for when they look at the ingredients portion of a food package.* The same IFIC surveys indicate that the top three concerns for older adults are type of fat or oil, type of sweetener, whether ingredients are natural, and the order of ingredients.

---

[5] *Deficit Reduction Act of 2005*, §6071, 6086, 6087.
[6] Available online: http://www.foodinsight.org/ (accessed August 5, 2010).

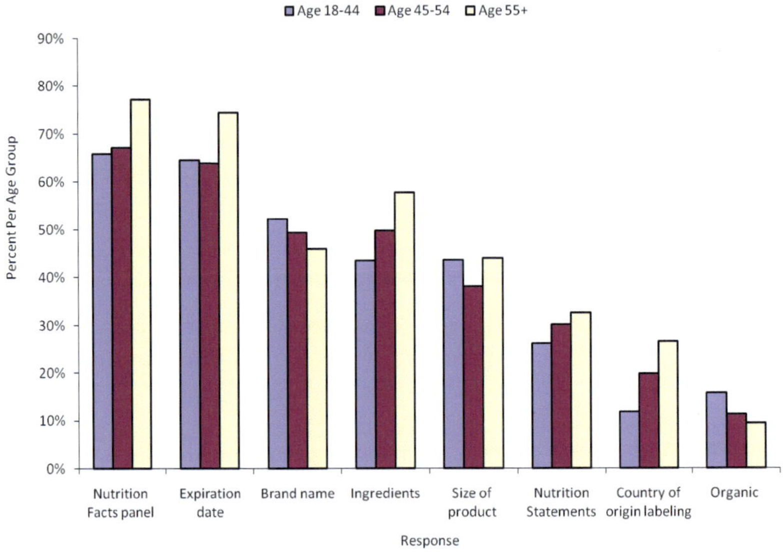

FIGURE 2-9 Food and beverage package information used by shoppers when deciding to purchase or eat a food or beverage.
NOTE: Survey respondents were asked "What information do you look for on the food or beverage package when deciding to purchase or eat a food or beverage? Check all that apply."
SOURCE: IFIC, 2009.

- *Whether shoppers 55 years and older have made a change based on hearing something about food, food safety, or nutrition in the news.* The IFIC surveys also revealed that about 60 percent of shoppers 55 years and older had heard or read something that prompted them to change their mind about a food purchase.

Food Preparation and Consumption Behavior

Wellman remarked that most of the data she would be sharing on food preparation and consumption behavior were proprietary data made available by the NPD Group, a Chicago-based market research company, and she thanked Suzie Crocket from General Mills for allowing her to access the data. Using a variety of sources, the NPD Group collects data on pantry preparation, individual consumption behavior, motivations and attitudes that drive people to eat the way they do, etc. Wellman focused on two categories of data: (1) "boomers without children": one- or two-member households without children (adults 44–62 years old) and (2) "matures": one- or two-member households without children (adults 63 years and older).

Preparation Behavior

Both boomers without children and matures spend less time overall preparing and cooking foods than families with children, with much less time spent preparing and cooking in the morning compared to later in the day. For example, both groups spend about 2 minutes preparing and another 2 minutes cooking their morning meals and about 12 minutes preparing and 25 minutes cooking their evening meals. For both groups, the number of dishes per meals is fairly small and increases as the day goes on. For example, not including beverages, both groups prepare and cook about 1.5 dishes for breakfast, 2 dishes for lunch, and 2.5 dishes for dinner.

Matures tend to eat more of their meals at home than boomers without children do, with breakfast being the meal most often eaten at home. For matures, breakfast is also generally considered the most satisfying in terms of nutritional quality. As people age, dinners tend to be aimed at meeting convenience needs, with less planning, less use of ovens, grills, or stovetops, greater use of appliances such as microwaves and toasters, (matures have the highest lunchtime appliance use, probably because more are retired and eat lunch at home) and less clean up. Because the goal is convenience, dinners tend to be not as satisfying from a nutritional quality standpoint.

Wellman briefly discussed IFIC survey data showing that while respondents ages 55 and older were a little more likely to regularly perform actions to ensure food safety when cooking, preparing, and consuming food products, there is room for improvement among respondents of all age groups in regularly performing these actions. In terms of microwavable meals, older adults are slightly more likely than other age groups to follow all cooking instructions, check the label for conditions of use, and let the food stand for an appropriate time after microwaving. Nonetheless, only 40–80 percent of respondents in all age groups reported regularly following any of those actions. As shown in Figure 2-10, all respondents, particularly those in the 18–44 year-old age group, reported a number of obstacles to safe food handling, all associated with a lack of something—information, time, proper equipment, or interest.

Consumption Habits

For both boomers without children and matures, most consumption choices are driven not by health but by convenience, taste, and indulgence. That said, according to NPD Group data, health is the most important driver in the morning, and it drives more food choices in general among matures (34 percent) than among boomers without children (27 percent). This may be because different moods affect food choices, and matures tend to be more relaxed, calm, and content than boomers without children.

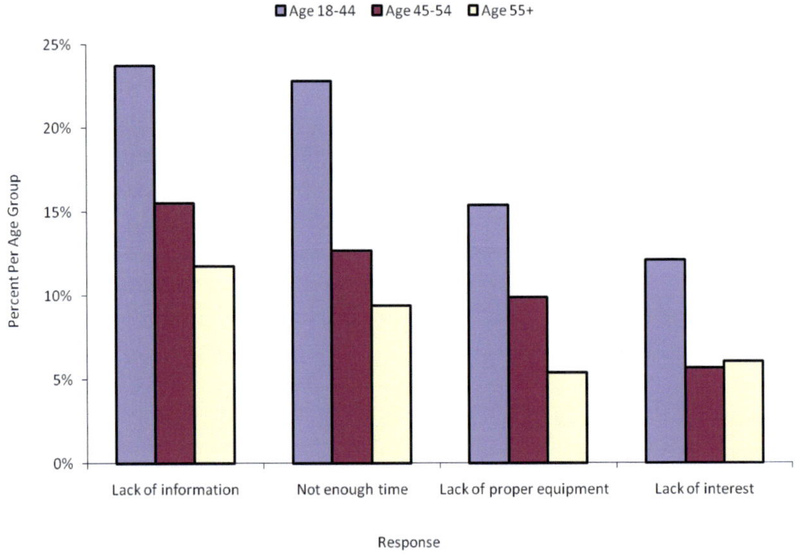

FIGURE 2-10 Obstacles survey respondents reportedly face when handling food safely.
NOTE: Survey respondents were asked, "What obstacles, if any, do you face when handling food safely? Check all that apply."
SOURCE: IFIC, 2009.

In terms of what people actually eat for breakfast at home, for both matures and boomers without children, juices and healthy ready-to-eat cereals rank fairly high (only coffee ranks higher than either). Other top choices include fruit, bread (toast, bagels, etc.), hot cereals, eggs and omelets, milk, hot tea, pancakes/waffles/French toast, bacon, carbonated soft drinks, and fruit drinks. Matures consume more fruit juice and hot cereal than boomers do.

For lunch at home, top foods and beverages include sandwiches, fruit, vegetables, carbonated soft drinks, milk, soup, tea, salads, salty snacks, coffee, and crackers. Matures tend to eat more vegetables, milk, soup, and coffee than boomers do.

For dinner at home, top food and beverage choices include vegetables, salads, potatoes, fruit, carbonated soft drinks, tea, sandwiches, poultry, milk, bread, beef, soup, coffee, and alcoholic beverages. Matures tend to eat more fruit at dinner than boomers do. Wellman noted that these choices do not look so bad, given that health drives only 1 in 10 dinner choices. Most dinner choices are driven by convenience (38 percent for boomers without children, 41 percent for matures) and personal preference and taste (34 percent for boomers, 31 percent for matures).

Everyone snacks, with indulgence driving about half of all snack choices. So even though many people do fairly well in terms of eating nutritiously at breakfast and lunch, they tend to snack on what they really like without much consideration for health. Only 8 percent of boomers and 9 percent of matures cited health as a driver of snack choices. Top snack foods include candy, fruits, nuts and seeds, ice cream, cookies, potato chips, crackers, pretzels, microwave popcorn, yogurt, tortilla chips, and ice cream bars. Matures tend to favor cookies, crackers, pretzels, and yogurt more than boomers do.

Overall and based on the Healthy Eating Index, matures tend to eat more healthfully than boomers without children do, although overall they could be eating even more healthfully. Thirty-eight percent of matures have "most healthful" eating habits, compared to 25 percent of boomers; 41 percent of matures have "moderately healthful" eating habits, compared to 44 percent of boomers; and 21 percent of mature have "least healthful" habits, compared to 31 percent of boomers (Figure 2-11).

Matures are more concerned with negative food attributes, such as salt, fat, and cholesterol, than boomers without children. For example, accord-

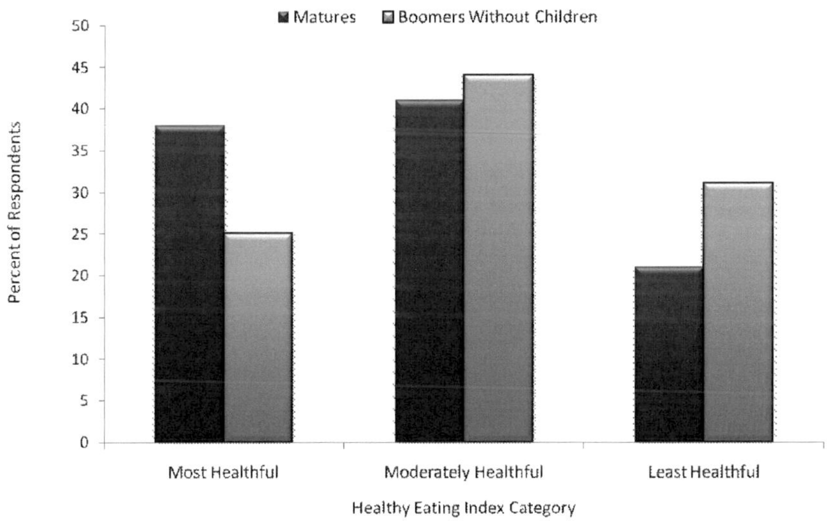

FIGURE 2-11 Percent of matures and boomers without children falling into three Healthy Eating Index categories.
NOTE: "Boomers without children" are defined as one- or two-member households without children (adults 44–62 years old). "Matures" are defined as one- or two-member households without children (adults 63 years and older).
SOURCE: NPD Group/Food and Beverage Services.

ing to NPD Group data, 70 percent of matures are concerned with total fat content, compared to 64 percent of boomers; 63 percent of matures are concerned with salt, compared to 61 percent of boomers; and 64 percent of matures are concerned with cholesterol, compared to 60 percent of boomers. Dieting, however, tends to decrease with age, with 25 percent of boomers and 21 percent of matures reporting that they were on a diet in one NPD Group survey.

Food Insecurity and Hunger

Based on USDA data (2009), Wellman described how food spending has decreased over the past several years—12 percent relative to the rising cost of the USDA Thrifty Food Plan[7] and 6 percent relative to the rising consumer price index (CPI) for food and beverages. The largest decline has been in the second lowest income quintile, where average CPI-inflation-adjusted spending for food decreased 16 percent. Median food spending among older adults living alone dropped 5.4 percent between 2000 and 2007. This decrease, coupled with the fact that one in six older adults already eats fewer than 1,000 calories a day, raises serious questions about food insecurity. Among older adults living alone, very low food security (i.e., hunger) increased 1 percent from 1.9 percent to 2.8 percent between 2000 and 2007.

Two research reports by Ziliak and colleagues (2008, 2009)[8] show that 11.4 percent of all seniors experienced some form of food insecurity between 2000–2005 because they did not have enough money. Of these, about 2.5 million were at risk of hunger, and 750,000 actually suffered from hunger due to financial constraints. These reports find that the risk of hunger is greatest among those with limited incomes (almost half of all older adults at risk of hunger are low income or below poverty), those under the age of 70, African-Americans and Hispanics, never-married individuals, renters, and people who live in the South. Together, the data indicate that food insecurity is a major problem, with Ziliak and colleagues predicting that by 2025, millions of older Americans will be facing hunger. By 2025, an estimated 9.5 million older Americans will be marginally food insecure, 3.9 million will be food insecure, and 1 million will be very low food secure.

---

[7] The Thrifty Food Plan is a USDA-developed national standard for a nutritious diet at minimal cost. It is based on average national food prices adjusted for inflation and is used as the basis for food stamp allotments.

[8] Available online: http://www.mowaa.org/Page.aspx?pid=654 (accessed August 27, 2010).

USDA Federal Nutrition Assistance Programs

Given this trend in food insecurity, Wellman argued that efforts to reduce hunger will need to be continued and strengthened. One way to do this is through federal nutrition assistance programs, many of which are USDA programs. Wellman briefly described these programs and suggested ways they could be improved:

- *Supplemental Nutrition Assistance Program (SNAP):* The good news, Wellman argued, is that President Obama has increased funding for SNAP to a total budget of $48 billion for fiscal year 2010. The bad news is that only 30 percent of older adults who are eligible participate, compared to 65 percent participation by the total eligible population. Of all food stamp participants, only 9 percent are older adults. Based on criteria set by the USDA Thrifty Food Plan, the monthly benefit for single older adults is lower ($74) than it is for younger adults (up to $100), so age is somewhat penalizing. Wellman suggested that the nutritionists and economists responsible for developing the USDA Thrifty Food Plan need to consider that homebound or bed-bound older adults may need more pre-prepared foods or convenience foods in order to eat more healthfully.
- *SNAP Education Program:* States have the option to provide nutrition guidance to accompany the SNAP Program, but the focus is on women and children, not older adults. Because older adults are generally seen as interested in improving their food and nutritional intake, Wellman suggested that they would probably listen to the advice. This is particularly true given that they are receiving less money than younger adults and therefore need more help using that money wisely.
- *Commodity Supplemental Food Program:* Perhaps surprisingly, 93 percent of participants in this program are older adults (i.e., 444,000 older adults participate, compared to 31,000 other people). However, the quantities of food packages provided in the commodity boxes are often impractical for one- or two-person households. Although USDA has been making some changes to the quality and quantity of food offered through this program, additional improvements could be made.
- *The Emergency Food Assistance Program:* Because this is an emergency program, it cannot be considered a hallmark of federal efforts to reduce food insecurity; and although it is intended to supplement low-income, in-need individuals, including older adults, states set the criteria. Moreover, the commodity foods are not sent directly to

individuals but rather are sent to local distributing agencies, such as food banks and soup kitchens, which do not always prioritize older adults. Wellman noted that sensitivity to older adult needs among local distributing agents must be improved.

- *Senior Farmers' Market Nutrition Program:* Forty-three states and seven tribes have this program in place. However, it is available only during the local growing season; and the budget is very small. The average benefit per person is only $23 per year, or approximately $2 per month. (During the discussion session following this presentation, a member of the audience commented that the program provides $20.6 million annually through 2012 and that states that receive grants are required to provide nutrition education.)
- *Child and Adult Care Food Program (CACFP):* Intended primarily for children, disabled adults, and older adults in non-residential day centers, this program is state-regulated with no data available on older adult participation. Wellman described a new Institute of Medicine (IOM) Food and Nutrition Board consensus study under way, which will review and assess the nutritional needs of the target populations and make meal requirement recommendations for the CACFP.

U.S. Department of Health and Human Services Federal Nutrition Assistance

The largest federal nutrition assistance program for older adults is the Older Americans Act (OAA) Nutrition Program, operated by the U.S. Department of Health and Human Services Administration on Aging. The purpose of the program, which is popularly known as "Meals on Wheels" and "Senior Dining," is to reduce hunger and food insecurity, promote socialization of older individuals, and promote the health and well-being of older individuals. Unlike the USDA programs, it has no income requirements and forbids means testing. Although the program targets individuals in greatest economic and social need, low-income minorities, and people living in rural areas, the only real criterion is that a participant be more than 60 years of age. Because states drive the program, with minimal federal regulations and minimal uniformity, there is considerable variation in how the program operates across the country.

One of the problems with the program is its limited nutrition capacity and technical assistance. There is only one national nutritionist, only one regional nutritionist (in New England), no nutritionists in 55 percent of the state-level units on aging, and no national nutrition resource center.

The program reaches about 2.6 million older adults, serving about 241 million meals annually. Most of these are home-delivered, but about a third are congregate meals served to senior centers, etc. Overall, the number of home-delivered meals is increasing—about 61 percent of OAA meals served in 2008 were delivered to the home, reaching 909,913 older adults. That amounts to 161 meals per participant. Wellman said, "If we are going to keep people out of nursing homes, we probably could do a better job of providing more than 161 meals to people who are homebound." Total annual expenditure averaged $828 per participant—a figure, Wellman observed, that is equal to the cost of one day in the hospital. Also in 2008, 39 percent of total meals served were served as congregate meals, reaching 1,656,634 older adults (58 meals per participant), with the total annual expenditure averaging $384 per participant.

Forty-eight percent of older adults who receive homebound meal deliveries live alone, and 63 percent are female. Thirty-five percent of older adults who go to senior centers to eat meals live alone, and 63 percent are female. Even though people need be only 60 years of age to participate, the average age of OAA meal participants is about 74 to 75. About a third of the home-delivered participants are considered nursing home-eligible because of the number of disabilities they have. When asked, 93 percent of participants said that having one meal delivered five days a week allows them to stay home. For about 60 percent of older adults receiving meals either at home or in senior centers, that single meal comprises over half of their food intake for the day.

Wellman compared the OAA Nutrition Program with the Supplemental Nutrition Program for Women, Infants, and Children (WIC), both of which started at about the same time. The OAA Nutrition Program had a budget of $125 million its first year (1974), and WIC had a budget of $20.6 million (1975). In 2008, the OAA program's budget was $784 million, compared to WIC's $6.2 billion. Appropriations for the older adult program have grown only six-fold, whereas funds for WIC have grown 332-fold. One of the reasons for this discrepancy, Wellman argued, may be that outcomes for WIC have been documented from the very beginning, with a focus on nutrition. The OAA program is not as focused on outcomes.

A New Position Statement on Food and Nutrition Programs for Community-Dwelling Older Adults

Far too often, Wellman said, community food and nutrition programs for older adults are disregarded, taken for granted, or underfunded. Because of this, the American Dietetic Association (ADA), the American Society for Nutrition (ASN), and the Society for Nutrition Education (SNE) developed a position statement on food and nutrition programs for community-dwelling older adults (Kamp et al., 2010):

- Given the federal cost containment policy to rebalance long-term care away from nursing homes to home and community based services, it is the position of ADA, ASN, and SNE that all older adults should have access to food and nutrition programs that ensure the availability of safe, adequate food to promote optimal nutrition status.
- Appropriate food and nutrition programs include adequately funded nutrition assistance and meal programs, nutrition education, screening, assessment, counseling, therapy, monitoring, evaluation, and outcomes documentation to assure healthier aging.
- The growing number of older adults, the health care focus on prevention, and the global economic situation accentuate the fundamental need for these programs.

In closing, Wellman said that the position statement essentially states that the trend in the United States is toward community living and keeping older adults out of institutional settings. Given this situation, the position statement encourages the intensification of efforts to feed older adults at home.

QUESTIONS AND DISCUSSION

Kinsella and Wellman's talks prompted questions about data on poverty and aging, the relationship between obesity and longevity, and the trend among aging populations toward increased community living (and assisted living) and away from nursing home living.

Poverty and Aging

The first question pertained to Kinsella's data showing a decline over time in poverty among older adults, whereas Wellman's data showed an increase in hunger among older adults as a result of increased poverty. The questioner asked how these seemingly contradictory trends should be interpreted. Kinsella explained that while the percentage of older adults in poverty has decreased, the absolute number of older adults in poverty has increased and is still significantly high. Wellman agreed and explained that the data she presented were from a report prepared for Congress and that the figures were represented in actual numbers (i.e., millions of people), not percentages.

The Relationship Between Obesity and Longevity

There was another question about Kinsella's data showing an increase over time in longevity, even though some experts have predicted a decline in longevity because of obesity. Kinsella replied, "That's the 64 million dollar question right now." He stated that the relationship between obesity and mortality is not well established and that while intuitively it makes sense, so far there is remarkably little scientific evidence showing that in fact obesity is related to mortality. Another audience member remarked that while obesity may not be directly associated with mortality, there are quite robust data showing an association between obesity and functional decline with aging, including mobility impairments, and an increased risk of becoming homebound. He stated that in terms of quality of life and the ability to live independently, obesity is an important issue with respect to aging. The same audience member remarked that many obese older adults "may not be for want of food energy" but "eat such poor quality diets they are malnourished." He noted a very high prevalence of dietary and serum micronutrient deficiencies in obese community-dwelling elderly people. Chapter 3 includes a more detailed discussion of inadequate nutrient intakes among older adults.

The Trend Toward Community Living (and Assisted Living)

Another audience member asked about the trend toward not living in nursing homes: Where are people living, and does the OAA Nutrition Program deliver meals to assisted living facilities? Wellman explained that the program does not generally service assisted living facilities. However, she noted that meals could be provided at adult day centers, not necessarily by the OAA program but by the Child and Adult Care Food Program. She predicts that there will be a growing demand for adult day centers as efforts continue to be directed toward keeping older adults out of nursing homes and in the community.

Kinsella reiterated that the proportion of the older population residing in nursing homes or institutional residences has declined over the last 20 years or so, with a corresponding rise in the proportion of people living in assisted living facilities. However, there are many forms and gradations of assisted living, making it difficult to lump them all together and identify trends. With respect to the trend toward living alone, he noted that 40 percent of older women live alone. While some people interpret this as an "epidemic of isolation" and something to be concerned about, living alone may be more a function of being able to afford living alone rather than a reflection of social isolation. Older women today are much more likely to have some sort of social security or pension income than they did decades ago, and surveys have shown that if given a choice most people would like to spend as much of their life as possible at home. For Kinsella, the trend toward living alone and with the help of programs like the OAA Nutrition Program is a positive, not negative, sign.

Finally, an audience member remarked that the IOM Food and Nutrition Board has developed a proposal and is searching for sponsors for a future workshop on food and nutrition services for older adults.

3

Physiology and Aging

The session opened with moderator Gordon Jensen of Pennsylvania State University, University Park, Pennsylvania, remarking on the challenge of differentiating between aging and the multitude of chronic diseases that accompany aging. He then introduced the first of three speakers, Simin Nikbin Meydani of the Jean Mayer U.S. Department of Agriculture (USDA) Human Nutrition Research Center on Aging (HNRCA) at Tufts University, Boston, Massachusetts, who spoke about changes in the immune system that accompany aging and the importance of considering underlying genetic variation in immunity when evaluating nutrition in aging populations. Meydani emphasized the distinction between incidence of infectious disease and severity of illness resulting from infection. Meydani also presented evidence from a series of recent studies demonstrating how macro- and micro-nutritional supplementation can compensate for some of the immunological changes that accompany aging. Jensen himself then spoke about the gastrointestinal (GI) system and how it remains largely unchanged with aging, with most major changes being related to underlying conditions. He emphasized, however, that oral health is one component of the GI system that does typically decline with aging, with many older adults suffering from poor diet quality and micronutrient deficiencies as a result. Finally, Marcia Pelchat of the Monell Chemical Sciences Center, Philadelphia, Pennyslvania, discussed food-related sensory perception changes with age and the consequences of these changes.

IMMUNE STATUS OF AGING POPULATIONS AND METHODS OF MODULATING SUSCEPTIBILITY

Presenter: Simin Nikbin Meydani

Meydani began by commenting on how scientists have recently learned that dysregulation of immune and inflammatory response with aging not only contributes to greater susceptibility to infectious diseases and cancer, but also greater susceptibilities to other chronic diseases such as cardiovascular disease, Alzheimer's disease, osteoporosis, and type 2 diabetes. She remarked that most of her talk, however, would focus on the former: how dysregulation of the immune and inflammatory systems, most of which is associated with changes in T-cell-mediated function, contribute to an increasing incidence of infectious diseases and cancer with aging.

Aging and Infectious Diseases

Aging is associated with a higher incidence of morbidity and mortality from a number of different types of infectious diseases (e.g., pneumonia, tuberculosis, GI infections, urinary tract infections, and *Herpes zoster*). For example, pneumonia and influenza together are the fourth leading cause of death among older adults. Even when a diagnosis is cardiovascular disease, the cause of death is often pneumonia. While the incidence of GI infections is not necessarily any greater in the elderly population, morbidity and mortality from GI infections is much higher in older adults. For example, when a food poisoning episode occurs in a nursing home, the younger caregivers can usually recover, but the elderly people often suffer greater complications that may result in death.

To illustrate the impact that aging has on the severity of infectious disease, Meydani described a *Salmonella typhimurium* study that she and her colleagues conducted using a murine model system (Ren et al., 2009). They examined colonization of *Salmonella* after both young and old mice had been exposed to *Salmonella*. While in the beginning (one day post-infection), the young animals showed a higher colonization rate, the older animals showed a much higher colonization rate as their infections progressed (2–4 days post-infection). This was true at both low and high doses of exposure. Even early on, when the colonization rates were higher in the younger animals, the older animals nonetheless experienced greater weight loss because of the severity of the infection.

Meydani emphasized that the last observation is important to consider in relation to food safety because often efforts are directed toward preventing exposure to foodborne infectious agents without enough consideration about whether and how host response to infection could be improved to make older adults less susceptible to morbidity and mortality resulting from an infection once it does take hold.[1] Meydani gave several reasons that might explain why susceptibility to infectious disease increases with age:

- *Impaired immune response*, which occurs mostly because of changes in T cell-mediated functions. For example, in the same murine system previously described, Meydani and colleagues found that production of Interferon (IFN)-g is the same in young and old uninfected mice but that young infected animals show a significantly greater production of IFN-g than old infected animals. These results suggest that younger animals are more capable of mounting an effective immune response against *Salmonella typhimurium*. In humans, any of a number of T cell-mediated functions could be contributing to the link between aging and infectious diseases (as well as between aging and cancer), including decreased antibody production, a decreased delayed-type hypersensitivity (DTH) response, an increase in the percentage of memory cells and corresponding decrease in the percentage of naïve cells (thereby decreasing an individual's ability to respond to new infections), a decrease in the number of T-helper cells, etc. In addition to changes in the T cells themselves, other changes such as increased macrophage production of various suppressive factors can also lead to a decline in T cell-mediated function.
- *Increased pathogen virulence in aged hosts*. For example, Meydani described work by Melinda Beck, University of North Carolina, and colleagues on the coxsackie B3 (CVB3) virus. There are two types of CVB3 virus: one avirulent (CVB3/0 does not cause disease), the other virulent (CVB3/20 can cause myocarditis in animals and is known to be associated with Keshan disease, a cardiomyopathy associated with dietary deficiencies in selenium [Se]). Beck and colleagues showed that the avirulent version injected into Se-deficient mice will evolve into the virulent version (Beck et al., 1994). When the researchers separated the virus from the host and injected it back into another young animal that was not Se-deficient, the latter animal nonetheless developed myocarditis, suggesting that the normally mild virus had somehow become virulent in the Se-deficient mice. When the researchers sequenced the virus, they found mutations that resembled those of the virulent form. Suspecting that perhaps the

[1] Steven Gendel also elaborated on the distinction between incidence of foodborne infection and the severity of the consequences of infection during his presentation later in the workshop, as summarized in Chapter 4.

change was associated with increased oxidative stress in the Se-deficient animals, the researchers questioned whether they might find the same phenomena on mice similarly stressed in other ways. Indeed, they showed the same occurrence in animals fed diets deficient in vitamin E. Meydani and her colleagues wondered if the same might be true of aging, given that aging is also known to be associated with an increase in oxidative stress. So they did a similar passage experiment where they injected avirulent virus into both young and old animals (Gay et al., 2006). As expected, the young animals had low titers (i.e., little infection). However, the old animals not only showed higher titers but also more pathology and even some mortality. After avirulent strain was injected into old animals and then back into the young animals, suddenly the previously healthy young animals developed high titers, high pathology, and this virus exhibited numerous base changes in its nucleotide sequences, which made it similar to the virulent strain. These observations suggested that, as with a Se-deficient diet, there is something about the aging host that caused a normally mild virus to become virulent. So in addition to immunological changes that occur with aging, which make older individuals more susceptible to infection or more severe infections, unknown changes in the host environment might also be causing mutations that make pathogens more virulent.

- *Changes in gut microflora.* A limited number of studies (e.g., Hopkins and Macfarlane, 2002) have shown that structural changes can occur in the gut that result in a decrease in the number and diversity of beneficial bacteria (e.g., bifidobacteria) and a corresponding increase in the number and diversity of harmful bacteria (e.g., clostridia, enterobacteria). The reason for this change is unclear, although Meydani speculated that perhaps the same type of evolutionary change that the CVB3 virus appears to undergo could be occurring with bacteria as well.
- *Genetics and other physiological changes.* Differences in genetic background may be related to variation in response to nutritional interventions as described in the next section on nutrition supplementation. Meydani also suggested that micronutrient status in older adults could be a determinant of susceptibility to infectious disease.

Taken together, all of these changes that occur with aging raise the question: Can something be done to prevent age-associated immune dysfunction and/or viral evolution? What is the role of nutrition?

The Effect of Nutrient Supplementation on Susceptibility to Infectious Disease

For the remainder of her talk, Meydani described a series of studies on how supplementation with various micronutrients (vitamin E, zinc, vitamin B_6), macronutrients (fish oil), and caloric restriction can impact susceptibility to infectious disease. Meydani argued that taken together, all of this evidence suggests that nutritional manipulation can decrease susceptibility to infections in older adults.

Vitamin E

In a double-blind, placebo-controlled study, Meydani and colleagues demonstrated that supplementation with vitamin E can significantly improve immune response, particularly T cell-mediated response, in healthy older adults (Meydani et al., 1997). Meydani and colleagues fed healthy older adults different levels of vitamin E for six months and then examined, as an indication of immune response, the participants' abilities to produce antibodies against hepatitis B, tetanus toxoid, and pneumococcal vaccine, as well as *in vivo* cell-mediated immunity. At the workshop, she shared only the results relating to changes in antibody response to hepatitis B. All three vitamin E-fed groups (60, 200, and 800 international units [IU]), but particularly the 200 IU group, showed an increase in both antibody response and DTH diameter. The 200 IU group showed a 19.9 U/ml antibody response (compared to 3.3 U/ml in the control group) and a 65 percent change in DTH diameter of induration (compared to 18 percent among controls). Pallast et al. (1999) confirmed the findings.

Meydani and colleagues asked whether this improved immune response from vitamin E supplementation is also associated with an actual decrease in susceptibility to infection. They conducted another double-blind, placebo-controlled study (Meydani et al., 2004). Based on a year's worth of data from 617 nursing home residents, they found that older adults supplemented with vitamin E had significantly lower risk of acquiring upper but not lower respiratory infections. Upper respiratory infections tend to be viral, whereas lower respiratory infections tend to be bacterial.

However, in these various studies, not all of the older adults who received vitamin E supplementation showed improvements in immune response. There were responders and non-responders. Meydani and colleagues speculated that some of this variability may be due to genetic differences among the older adults. Knowing that host genetics influence cytokine production, they wondered if variation in cytokine genetics in particular could explain variability in response to vitamin E. Indeed, Belisle et al. (2009) found that vitamin E supplementation did not have a significant effect on tumor necrosis factor (TNF)-α production in individuals with a G/G genotype (TNF-α-308G>A) but significantly reduced TNF-α production in individuals with an A/G or A/A genotype. Meydani said that, interestingly, people with an A/G or A/A genotype normally produce a higher level of TNF-α, and vitamin E supplementation appears to be effective at reducing cytokine production only in individuals with initially high levels of cytokine.

Zinc

Also in Meydani et al. (2004), Meydani and colleagues measured the blood levels of various other micronutrients, including zinc. They were surprised to find that 30 percent of the participants were deficient in zinc (i.e., defined as less than 70 µg/dL). Knowing that zinc has been shown to play an important role in resistance to pneumonia, they questioned whether there might be a relationship between serum zinc levels and pneumonia. Not surprisingly, in a subsequent study, they found that the incidence of pneumonia in older adults with adequate zinc serum levels was half of what it was among older adults with low zinc serum levels (Meydani et al., 2007). Individuals with adequate zinc levels who did develop pneumonia had illnesses of shorter duration, fewer antibiotic prescriptions, and shorter durations of antibiotic use. These associations suggest that zinc status could be an important determinant of susceptibility to pneumonia among older adults.

Meydani emphasized that so far she and her colleagues have detected only an association between zinc and pneumonia. The next step is to determine whether zinc supplementation in older adults with initially low serum zinc levels actually reduces the incidence of pneumonia. She also mentioned that this high level of zinc deficiency is not unique to nursing home residents; in another study, she and her colleagues found that 22 percent of independently living older adults had low serum zinc levels.[2]

Vitamin B_6

Meydani described a study that she conducted in collaboration with Rob Russell (Meydani et al., 1990) on the effect of vitamin B_6 depletion and supplementation on immune response in the elderly. They found that depletion results in a significant reduction of lymphocyte percentage and that supplementation partially reversed the downward trend. However, the final lymphocyte percentage was still significantly lower than the initial

[2] These data are unpublished from Rall and colleagues.

baseline value. In terms of functionality, for example with respect to the availability of lymphocytes for interleukin 2 production and lymphocyte proliferation, they observed the same pattern. Vitamin B_6 depletion was followed by significant reductions in both measures of functionality. Although supplementation partially reversed this trend, they were not able to bring the levels back up to what they were at baseline. Meydani explained that this inability to raise the levels to baseline could have been a function of the duration of supplementation (i.e., perhaps they needed to supplement for a longer period of time) and that the results nonetheless suggest that the status of vitamin B_6 is clearly important for healthy immune system functioning.

Fish Oil

Fish oil contains the n-3 polyunsaturated fatty acids, eicosapentaenoic acid (EPA), and docosahexaenoic acid (DHA).[3] Meydani explained that EPA has been shown to replace arachidonic acid (AA)[4] in membrane phospholipids in cells, thereby reducing the formation of pro-inflammatory lipids such as prostaglandin E_2 (PGE_2). Prostaglandins have been shown to have a suppressive effect on T cell function. Knowing that aging is associated with an increased production of PGE_2, Meydani and colleagues questioned whether a reduction in PGE_2 might have an impact—not just by reducing inflammation in older adults but also by affecting cell-mediated immunity. They conducted a study whereby they fed older adults with either a low-level fish oil diet (0.13 percent of calories) or a high-level fish oil diet (0.54 percent of calories) for six months and showed that, yes, diets enriched with fish-derived polyunsaturated fatty acids significantly reduced production of PGE_2 as well as production of the pro-inflammatory cytokines interleukin 1β, TNF, and interleukin 6 (Meydani et al., 1993). Surprisingly, in the same study, the researchers also found a significant reduction in DTH, which is not a desirable effect as DTH is an index of T cell-mediated function. They suspected that this adverse effect might be related to the increased need for antioxidant nutrients when consuming a high polyunsaturated fat diet. In a subsequent study, they showed that by consuming both supplemental fish oil and vitamin E in combination, older adults derive the beneficial anti-inflammatory effect of fish oil but without the adverse effect on T cell-mediated function that occurs when fish oil is administered alone (Wu et al., 2006) (see Figure 3-1).

---

[3] EPA and DHA are omega-3 fatty acids.

[4] AA is an omega-6 fatty acid.

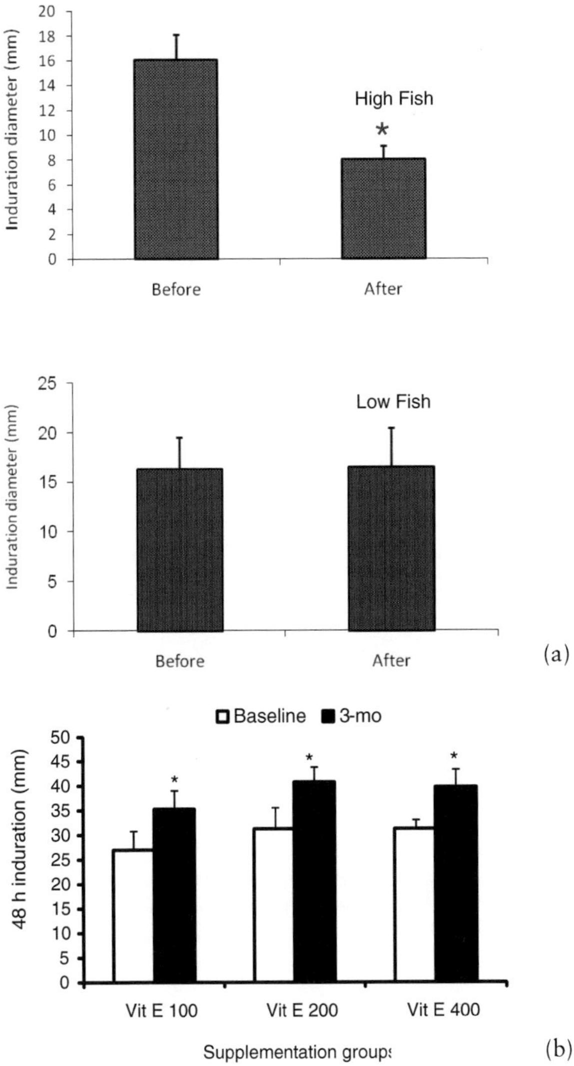

FIGURE 3-1 (a) When fish oil alone is administered to older adults, delayed-type hypersensitivity (DTH) levels decrease. (b) When administered in combination with vitamin E, DTH levels increase.
NOTE: (a) * = significantly different from before; (b) Mean ± SE, n = 8 to 10/group; $*p < 0.05$ compared to the baseline
SOURCES: Meydani et al., 1993; Wu et al., 2006.

Caloric Restriction

Finally, Meydani commented on a recent study on the effects of caloric restriction in humans. While there are plentiful data showing that caloric restriction can extend life in animals, data on its biological effects in humans are sparse.[5] Funded by the National Institute on Aging, CALERIE (Comprehensive Assessment of Long-Term Effects of Reducing Intake of Energy) is a multi-center study on the effects of 2 years of caloric restriction in humans. The Jean Mayer USDA HNRCA at Tufts University is one of the participating centers. Data collection was conducted in two phases. Meydani described results from the first (pilot) phase (Hayek et al., 1994). The design was randomized, controlled, and single-blinded; the participants were men and women between the ages of 25 and 45 and with a body mass index between 25 and 29 kg/m^2 (evidence suggests that the earlier caloric restriction is started, the more effective it will be); participants were exposed to either 10 percent or 30 percent reduced calorie diets; and DTH was used as an indicator of immune response and measured at both baseline and after 6 months. Among other findings, the study showed that both the 10 percent and 30 percent reduced calorie diets led to significant improvements in immune responses based on DTH measurements. Both diets also led to significant increases in concanavalin A and phytohemagglutinin-induced lymphocyte proliferation. However, only the 30 percent reduced calorie diet was effective at increasing anti-CD3-induced lymphocyte proliferation levels and reducing PGE_2 production.

Meydani cautioned that while the data suggest that caloric restriction could be effective in humans, this does not necessarily mean that caloric restriction "is good for the frail elderly." Participants in that study were between the ages of 25 and 45 and slightly overweight. She said that caloric restriction might, however, be beneficial in older adults who are overweight.

Conclusion

In conclusion, Meydani listed other dietary components that have been shown to be effective in improving or having some impact on the immune response in older adults: glutathione, conjugated linoleic acid, mushroom-derived glycopolysaccharide, and probiotics.

---

[5] For more detailed discussion on other recent studies on the effect of caloric restriction on aging, see the summary of Luigi Fontana's presentation in Chapter 5.

GASTROINTESTINAL SYSTEM CHANGES WITH AGE

Presenter: Gordon Jensen

Jensen began by commenting on the fact that there has not been much recent research on GI function in aging, probably because GI function is largely preserved over time in healthy adults—most dysfunction is an indication of an underlying condition. The remainder of his talk was an overview of the changes that occur along the GI tract with aging, beginning with the oropharynx and ending with the colorectum. The most important clinically relevant changes that occur in healthy older adults are in the oropharynx, with poor oral health being associated with poor diet quality, micronutrient deficiencies, involuntary weight loss, and an increased risk of cardiovascular disease.

Oropharynx

Some of the most important changes that occur with aging and that impact nutritional status occur in the oropharynx. Teeth become stained and worn and their roots become fragile and susceptible to fracture; and periodontal disease and tooth loss are common. In fact, many older adults are edentulous (without teeth) and without dental care insurance or entitlement programs for dental care. Many older adults also lack or have poor-fitting dentures. Other oropharyngeal changes known to occur with aging include swallowing dysfunction (15 percent of community-dwelling older adults have reported concerns); reduction in mastication and tongue muscle mass; dry mouth (40 percent of older persons complain of this) and decreased saliva production (which is usually caused by medical conditions, medications, or dehydration); delay in pharyngeal swallowing and decreased peristaltic amplitude and velocity; impairment of the laryngeal swallowing reflex; and a modestly increased risk of aspiration (which can lead to aspiration pneumonia).

Jensen and colleagues have found that the persistence of oral health problems in older adults is associated with various comorbidities (e.g., diabetes, obesity), impaired diet health quality (as measured by the Healthy Eating Index), and micronutrient deficiencies (Bailey et al., 2004). Citing work by Dennis Sullivan at the University of Arkansas, Little Rock, and colleagues, he stated that oral health problems are also known to be associated with significant involuntary weight loss in older adults (Sullivan et al., 1993). Periodontal disease in particular is also known to be associated with an increased risk of cardiovascular disease, probably because it reflects what Jensen described as a "smoldering inflammatory state." He explained that individuals with periodontal disease often have elevated C-reactive protein levels and that this same inflammatory state probably also injures the vascular endothelium and predisposes affected individuals to an increased risk of cardiovascular disease.

Esophagus

Significant impairment in the esophagus (i.e., impaired motility) usually reflects an underlying disease or condition, such as the presence of a tumor. Aging itself typically is associated with only more modest change, with many older adults showing decreased upper and lower sphincter pressures, reduced amplitude of peristaltic contractions, incomplete sphincter relaxation, delayed esophageal emptying, frequent tertiary contractions, esophageal dilation, and decreased neurons in the myenteric plexus. Unless there is an underlying disease or condition, these changes are usually not clinically symptomatic.

Stomach

While gastric acid secretion (both basal and stimulated) is generally well preserved in older adults, about one-third of older adults have atrophic gastritis (chronic inflammation of the stomach mucosa) and associated hypochlorhydria or achlorhydria (little or no gastric acid production, respectively). Atrophic gastritis is associated with a loss of gastric folds. Non-steroidal anti-inflammatory drugs (NSAID) gastropathy is even more common than atrophic gastritis, not just because of increased NSAID use among older adults but also because of impaired mucosal defense mechanisms in the aging stomach. Finally, gastric emptying tends to become delayed with mixed or solid meals but not with liquid meals, although a clinically significant delay usually reflects an underlying disease condition (e.g., diabetes).

Liver

The liver decreases in size with aging as a consequence of reduced hepatocyte regeneration. Blood flow to the liver declines as well. These changes result in a reduced capacity to metabolize many drugs, which has important implications for drug dosing in older adults. Aging livers also often demonstrate increased expression of inflammation-related genes. However, liver function tests are generally well preserved with the exception of albumin synthesis, which tends to decrease slightly. But it is difficult to attribute the change in albumin synthesis to aging alone because any smoldering inflammatory state could also induce the same change. Reduced albumin levels are better indicators of an underlying inflammatory state or chronic disease condition, and generally are not valid indicators of nutritional status.

Pancreas

The weight of the pancreas decreases with aging, with increased ductal epithelial hyperplasia leading to a narrowing of the ducts and lobular fibrosis. However, as with other GI organs and despite decreases in trypsin and lipase, the exocrine functions of the pancreas remain adequate unless there is some underlying serious disease (e.g., chronic pancreatitis). While decreased insulin secretion has been demonstrated in aging rodents, it is not clear whether this is true of humans. It conceivably could play a role in late-onset diabetes.

Small Intestine

As with most other sections of the GI tract, significant alterations in small bowel motility, transit, or function likely reflect underlying disease. The structure and absorptive functions of the small intestine are generally well preserved with aging. Small intestine surface area, crypt depth, villous height, enterocytes, and brush border show little change, and brush border enzyme activity for glucose transport is well maintained. While lactase activity declines, sucrase and maltase activities are unaffected. By and large, small intestinal integrity remains largely intact in healthy older adults, with normal mannitol absorption measurements.[6]

While decreased nutrient absorption is exhibited with aging, Jensen reiterated that significant changes in absorption of any nutrient usually reflect an underlying pathology.

High on the list of nutrients with decreased absorption levels is vitamin B_{12}, which Jensen explained is often a result of achlorhydria. Others include lactose, calcium, vitamin D (which shows a decrease in active transport as well as a decrease in receptors), iron, zinc, and magnesium. On the other hand, most macronutrients (protein, fat, and carbohydrate) and some vitamins (riboflavin and vitamin B_6) exhibit little change in absorption. Absorption of vitamin A increases with aging.

Colorectum

Unlike most other sections of the GI tract, the large bowel undergoes some significant structural changes with aging. These include increased collagen, elastic, elaunin, and oxytalan fibers; and decreased neuronal density. Postprandial augmentation of mass movements and segmented contractions of the colon, on the other hand, usually change only modestly, supporting a

[6] Mannitol is a common intestinal permeability probe. Malabsorption of mannitol is considered to be an indication of impaired functional integrity of the small intestine and of small intestinal diseases, such as celiac disease.

normal transit in most healthy older adults. However, certain dietary factors, diseases, medications (e.g., narcotics), and inactivity can nonetheless create significant clinical issues. In fact, self-reported constipation and laxative use increase with aging and are more prevalent among women. Other typical changes include an increased pressure threshold for eliciting a sense of rectal filling, decreased rectal elasticity, a thickening of the internal anal sphincter, and impairment in anal canal resting and maximal squeeze pressures. While older adults, especially women, report an increased frequency of fecal incontinence, this is usually associated with colorectal surgery or disease.

Microbiota

Again, GI microbiota appear to be relatively stable throughout adult life. Measurable changes are usually attributable to changes in diet, changes in GI function, or changes in the host immune system. Jensen cited Woodmansey (2007) and referred to Meydani's comments about studies that have shown an increase in the number and diversity of facultative anaerobes with aging and a corresponding decrease in the number and diversity of beneficial lactobacilli and bifidobacteria (Figure 3-2). Conceivably, this change in GI microbiota could lead to an increased risk of gastroenteritis and *Clostridium difficile* infection (which is an issue for hospitalized or chronic care facility patients who are administered antimicrobials that disrupt their normal bowel flora) and an increased risk of translocation of harmful bacteria.

Jensen remarked that there are a number of therapeutic strategies for intervening and favorably impacting altered microbiota (i.e., prebiotics,

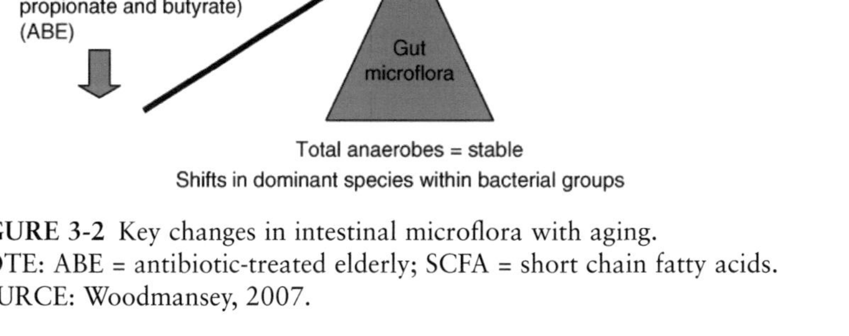

FIGURE 3-2 Key changes in intestinal microflora with aging.
NOTE: ABE = antibiotic-treated elderly; SCFA = short chain fatty acids.
SOURCE: Woodmansey, 2007.

probiotics, and synbiotics) and that our European colleagues "are probably at least a decade ahead of us in this very interesting area of research." Prebiotics are food ingredients that favor the growth of desirable bacteria (e.g., oligofructosaccharides). Probiotics are live microbial supplements (e.g., lactobacilli, bifidobacteria). Synbiotics are combinations of prebiotics and probiotics. Benefits have been reported (mostly from small, poorly controlled clinical trials) for the prevention of antibiotic-associated diarrhea, relapsing *C. difficile* colitis, traveler's diarrhea, and food-borne pathogen exclusion as well as the reduction of *H. pylori*-associated gastritis (McFarland, 2006, 2010).

Conclusion

In conclusion, Jensen emphasized the following:

- The aging GI system remains largely intact and functional.
- Clinical dysfunction usually reflects underlying disease or chronic conditions. Because absorptive functions remain intact in most healthy older adults, many nutritional supplements (e.g., those discussed during this workshop, such as vitamin E supplementation) are likely to be assimilated.
- Oral health in older adults, however, is a critical concern, with poor oral health leading to poor diet quality, micronutrient deficiencies, and involuntary weight loss.

SENSORY PERCEPTION CHANGES WITH AGING

Presenter: Marcia Pelchat

Pelchat presented an overview of the major taste, olfactory, and other food-related changes in sensory perception that typically occur with aging.

Age-Related Changes in Sense of Taste

Age-related loss of taste sensitivity is a well-known phenomenon, with the degree of sensory loss varying across compounds. Sensitivity to sweet is the most likely taste to be spared with aging, although even it can be affected. Most of the change in taste sensitivity that occurs with aging is not a consequence but rather a correlate of aging, due in part to commonly used medications, such as those for cardiovascular problems (e.g., see Schiffman, 2009). Consequently, much of the loss of taste that accompanies aging is potentially reversible through change either in medication or medication formulation.

Pelchat said that according to her Monell colleague Beverly Cowart, the most disturbing changes in sense of taste with aging are distortions and phantoms. Distortions are changes in the way a stimulus tastes when it is in the mouth, for example when a sweet food tastes bitter or metallic. Phantoms are persistent taste sensations that are present all the time. In some cases, distortions and phantoms are medication-related.

However, aging is almost never accompanied by a complete loss of taste. Pelchat explained that the sense of taste is "organized extremely redundantly," with three different cranial nerves serving the taste buds on the tongue. Rarely are all three nerves impacted. When a complete loss of taste does occur (e.g., as it can following head and neck radiation), it is devastating for the individual and makes it almost impossible to eat. With only a reduced sense of taste, eating is still possible.

Sense of Olfaction

Pelchat explained that while only a small number of taste qualities (i.e., about four to six) exist, individuals nonetheless experience "thousands upon thousands of different flavors" because of olfaction. Compared to taste, changes in olfaction are generally much more pronounced with aging. She said that the prevalence of presbyosmia (the diminution or loss of the sense of smell with aging) is "definitely the rule rather than the exception" (Cain and Stevens, 1989). For example, the National Geographic Smell Survey, a classic study conducted in the 1980s, demonstrated higher thresholds among older adults for several different odorants (Wysocki and Gilbert, 1989). National Geographic Magazine included a set of six scratch-and-sniff odor samples (both food and non-food stimuli: androstenone, amyl acetate, galaxolide, eugenol, mercaptans, and rose) in an issue of the magazine, eliciting 1.42 million respondents worldwide. The results are shown in Figure 3-3. This was followed by a smaller, scientifically recruited sample of around 25,000 individuals. The results were the same: As aging increased, ability to detect odor declined. Even above the detection threshold, odors become less intense with aging. The data also showed gender differences, with men experiencing more olfactory loss than women.

Also, very importantly and as Pelchat and colleagues subsequently demonstrated (2001), not only does the rate of loss vary across odorants, but it also varies among individuals, particularly among the "young elderly." For example, one person might show an early decline in his or her sensitivity to vanilla but not rose, while somebody else shows the opposite. This makes it difficult to increase odorants in foods in order to make them more palatable. Pelchat stated that over the age of 80, however, sensitivity to odors

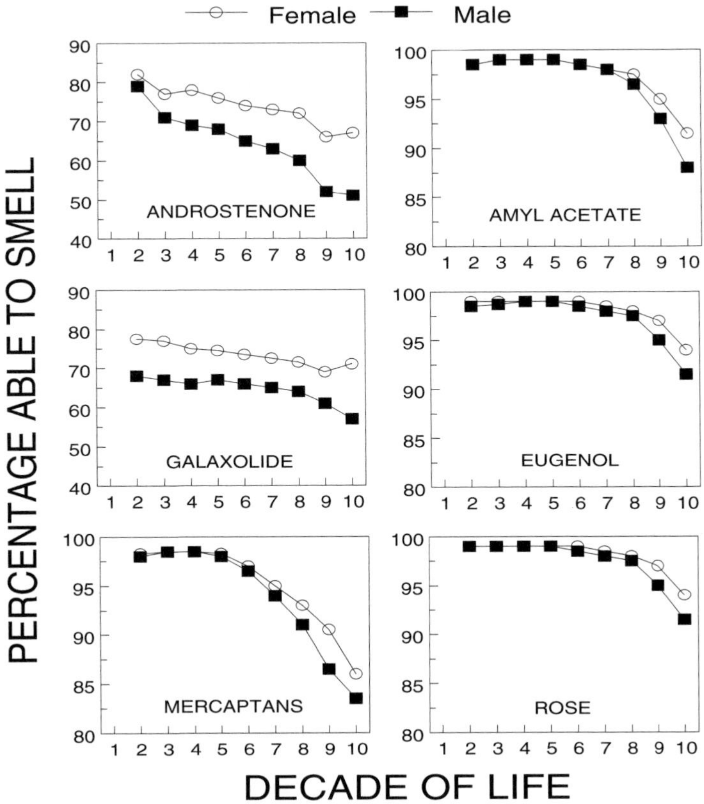

FIGURE 3-3 Comparison of an older population's ability to smell six different compounds.
SOURCE: Wysocki and Gilbert, 1989.

tends to decline "across the board," making it a little easier to increase palatability through odorant supplementation.

In a more recent epidemiological study, the Beaver Dam Study, which was mostly focused on hearing but also involved collecting olfactory data, over 60 percent of the people involved in the study over the age of 80 years had impaired sense of smell, and close to 25 percent of people over the age of 50 years were affected (Murphy et al., 2002). For Pelchat, one of the most important findings from that study was that self-report values dramatically underestimated the degree of loss (when compared to laboratory measures) (Shu et al., 2009). That is, when asked about their sense of smell, most older adults respond "it is just fine." Indeed, when the change is gradual, many people are not even aware of it.

In sum, although both aging-related loss of taste and smell vary across compounds and individuals, loss of olfactory sensitivity is more pronounced than loss of gustatory sensitivity.

The Sense of "Chemical Feeling"

There is a third food-related sense, which Pelchat said is sometimes referred to as "chemical feeling." It is the desirable irritation produced by carbonation and spices (e.g., chili pepper, ginger, and cinnamon) and which is not detected by the gustatory or olfactory systems but by a part of the nervous system more closely related to the skin senses. Pelchat explained that the same types of nerve endings that indicate when something hot has touched your cheek or that a foreign object is in your eye also innervate inside the nose and mouth and detect these "desirable irritants."

So far, there is no evidence for a decline in chemical feeling with age. For example, with carbonation, Pelchat and her group found that sensitivity (intensity of feeling) increased with increasing concentrations of carbonation, and that they did so for all age groups (young, middle-aged, and elderly).[7] In fact, elderly participants showed the greatest increase in intensity of feeling at the highest carbonation concentration levels. It is not clear why this is the case. There may be age-related changes in the oral mucosa that make it easier for these irritants to access the nerve endings.

Pelchat said that preservation of the sense of chemical feeling with aging could be perceived as either "good" or "bad." On one hand, for baby boomers who enjoy eating spicy Mexican or Thai food, it could serve as a form of oral stimulation that can be used to replace some of the other sensory losses. On the other hand, most flavorings are combinations of odorants, tastes, and irritants, and therefore adding more irritant can have an unpleasant burning effect unless the intensities of other flavor compounds are increased as well.

Most Older Adults Enjoy Eating

Despite chemosensory losses, most older adults nonetheless enjoy eating. While in the event of an upper respiratory infection or under other circumstances, chemosensory changes can be sudden and noticeable, most chemosensory loss with normal aging is gradual and undetectable. People compensate in unnoticeable ways, for example by leaving teabags to steep for longer periods of time. Pelchat and her colleagues have demonstrated that it is difficult to identify people with severe olfactory losses if they are eating familiar foods. For example, people who know that they are eating pear puree will say that what they are eating tastes like pear. But if they don't

[7] These data are unpublished from Pelchat.

know that they are eating a pear puree, they are very likely to misidentify the pear taste. This suggests that when people are in control of their purchase and preparation of food, their chemosensory losses may not have much effect. But if they are in a nursing home and eating a pureed diet without visual or textural cues, they may not know what they are eating.

Loss of Gate-Keeping Function

Pelchat said that importantly, a decreased intensity of flavor causes a shift toward something known as hedonic neutrality: pleasant flavors become less pleasant and unpleasant flavors become less unpleasant. Because of something known as negativity bias, people pay more attention to harmful experiences than to potentially beneficial experiences. So the effect of chemosensory loss is much greater for unpleasant flavors, which leads to a potential loss in what are known as gate-keeping functions, for example the ability to detect spoiled food or salt. Pelchat described the results of a study demonstrating that older adults living in institutionalized settings prefer saltier foods than younger adults living in the community, because of a loss in gate-keeping function (Figure 3-4).[8]

Conclusion

In summary, Pelchat emphasized the following:

- The elderly experience declines in sensitivity of all the chemical senses.
- Olfactory sensitivity declines the most.
- Most older adults are not aware of their loss of chemosensitivity.
- Loss of chemosensitivity is especially hard to detect in community-living elderly.
- Loss of chemosensitivity leads to a loss in gate-keeping functions.

QUESTIONS AND DISCUSSION

The three presentations sparked questions from the audience on vitamin E supplementation, differences in physiology between the 65-and-over and 85-and-over populations, the gate-keeping function of the mouth, epigenetics and the reality that aging is a lifetime process, and the association between loss of smell and Alzheimer's disease and other dementias.

[8] These data are unpublished from Pelchat.

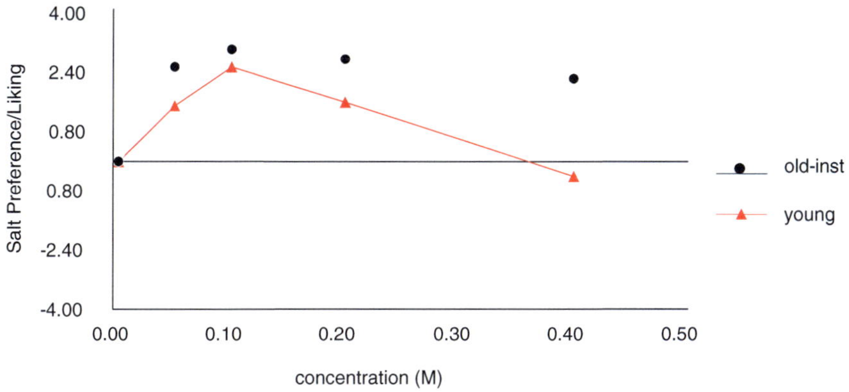

FIGURE 3-4 Loss in olfactory sensitivity with aging typically leads to a loss of gate-keeping function, with one of the manifestations being a decreased ability to detect salt.
SOURCE: Pelchat, unpublished data, 1993.

Vitamin E Supplementation

The first two questions were directed to Meydani, with the questioner asking about the benefits of vitamin E in middle-aged vs. older adults and the connection between vitamin E and omega-3 supplementation. Meydani explained that most of her studies have been with older adults. She recalled only one study involving both younger and older adults, which demonstrated some improvement in the younger adults but not to the degree seen in the older adults. Additionally, many animal model studies have shown that the benefit is greater for older ages. Without further studies in young adults, she said that she would be hesitant to recommend vitamin E supplementation to adults below the age of 50. With regard to the connection between vitamin E and fish oil, she said that most of those studies were done nearly 30 years ago, when there was considerable interest in fish oil. Both animal (rodent, primate) and human studies showed that fish oil must be combined with vitamin E in order to avoid the adverse effects associated with cell-mediated immunity. She said that the requirement for vitamin E is likely dependent on the type of fatty acid supplement.

Physiological Differences Among Different Older Age Groups

An audience member asked whether there are any differences in physiology between the 65-and-over versus 85-and-over populations. Most reports lump all older adults together into the 65-and-over category, but is this appropriate? Should this lumping be split into 65-and-over and 85-

and-over categories? Jensen responded, "That is a terrific question." He said that, as a clinician, he has observed tremendous variation between "old older persons" and "young older persons." Of course there are exceptions, and genetic imperative makes a tremendous difference as well. He described the differences as a continuum, and said "Drawing a line in the sand at a particular age is very challenging." Meydani agreed and added that the degree of change in immune system dysfunction during aging depends to some extent on the decade of age, and that there are differences between people in their 60s, for example, and people in their 90s.

The Gate-Keeping Function of the Oral Cavity

Another audience member asked Pelchat to elaborate on the concept of gate-keeping. Pelchat described the mouth as "the guardian of the body." She explained, "When you eat, you are potentially taking things into the body. One of the functions of the mouth is evaluating those things. . . . If there is a deep freeze in this guardianship, there may be more risk for adverse outcomes." Meydani added that loss of regulatory capacity during aging seems to be a common theme for many different functions. For example, older adults are often not able to detect hydration in the mouth, and they are less able to develop a response to infection (e.g., by developing a fever).

Aging as a Lifetime Process

The presenters were asked if they had given any consideration to whether epigenetics plays a role in aging-related physiological change. Does variation in early-life exposure (e.g., place of birth, nutrition during formative years) mean that different people have different optimal diets later in life? If so, how might this impact public policy around nutrition in aging populations? Meydani replied, "That is an excellent question." She said that she is considering that question in her own research, specifically how nutrition during early fetal life and during childhood could impact the development of chronic and infectious diseases later in life. It raises an important point: aging is a lifelong process, not just something that occurs in old age.

Loss of Smell

The last question was about the association between loss of smell and Alzheimer's disease. Pelchat replied that there is a very good correlation between loss of smell and Alzheimer's (and, more controversially, other dementias as well), as many of the changes associated with Alzheimer's begin in parts of the olfactory cortex. Prospective studies have found that people with severe olfactory loss develop more memory deficits in general, even if they do not develop Alzheimer's *per se*. However, she noted, "it is much more common to have a loss of sense of smell than to have Alzheimer's!"

4

Food Safety Concerns for Aging Populations

Moderated by Kerry Dearfield of the U.S. Department of Agriculture (USDA), this session comprised four presentations followed by a panel discussion. Steven Gendel of the Food and Drug Administration's (FDA's) Center for Food Safety and Applied Nutrition (CFSAN), College Park, Maryland, provided an overview of foodborne pathogens considered the greatest risk to aging populations, emphasizing that susceptibility to infection and severity of symptoms resulting from infection vary with age, depending on the pathogen. Furthermore, the two factors (susceptibility to infection and severity of illness) are not necessarily linked and should be monitored separately. Bernadene Magnuson of Cantox Health Sciences International, Bridgewater, New Jersey, discussed the effects of dietary food contaminants on health during aging. She also discussed surprising findings on the adverse effects of two purportedly beneficial dietary supplements, soy and curcumin, in older adults and emphasized the need to collect more safety data on active ingredients in dietary supplements. Food Forum Chair Michael Doyle of the University of Georgia, Athens, provided an overview of food processing and formulation technologies designed to protect against pathogens and contaminants, emphasizing the potential benefits and market sustainability of some of the newer non-thermal physical processing technologies and chemical treatments. He suggested that there could be niche market opportunities for some of the technologies that are otherwise having a difficult time penetrating the general marketplace (e.g., irradiated food products might be more acceptable and could be marketed to older adults, who are especially at risk of infection from foodborne pathogens). Finally, Aaron Brody of Packaging/Brody, Inc., Duluth,

Georgia, described recent innovations in food packaging, emphasizing that one of the main roles of food packaging is to provide protection against microbiological contamination. To conclude the session, David J. Greenblatt of Tufts University School of Medicine, Boston, Massachusetts, joined the four speakers in a panel session. Greenblatt offered a different perspective than Magnuson's on the issue of nutrient-drug interactions.

PATHOGENS OF CONCERN

Presenter: Steven Gendel

Gendel began by remarking that he would be exploring in detail which pathogens are considered to be of concern to aging populations and why. He explained that there are two factors to consider when determining whether a pathogen is of concern: (1) the probability that a person will develop an illness, given a certain level of exposure; and (2) the severity of the consequences if an illness does develop. These two factors are not necessarily directly linked and must be considered separately.

International Discrepancies in Pathogens of Concern

Different countries and even different agencies within a country (i.e., in the United States, FDA and the Centers for Disease Control and Prevention [CDC]) list different foodborne pathogens as being of concern to aging populations:

- In the "Bad Bug Book," FDA's handbook of foodborne microbes,[1] 19 foodborne pathogens are listed, only 6 of which are identified as being of concern to older adults.
- CDC lists 12 foodborne pathogens, only 4 of which are identified as being of concern.
- The United Kingdom (UK) Health Protection Agency lists 11 foodborne pathogens, only 4 of which are identified as being of concern for aging populations.
- The New Zealand Food Safety Authority (NZFSA) lists 16 foodborne pathogens, only 3 of which are identified as being of concern for aging populations.

Gendel remarked that not only are the numbers of listed pathogens surprisingly low, but there are some remarkable differences among the

[1] Available online: http://www.fda.gov/Food/FoodSafety/FoodborneIllness/FoodborneIllness FoodbornePathogensNaturalToxins/BadBugBook/default.htm.

agencies with respect to which particular infectious agents are considered to be of concern to older adults. All four agencies list *Listeria monocytogenes*, *Salmonella*, and *E. coli* O157:H7 as being of concern for aging populations, and all four agencies note the possibility of greater severity of disease with *Salmonella* and *E. coli* O157:H7 infections in older adults. However, only NZFSA considers *Shigella* to be of particular concern to aging populations, and only FDA considers *Clostridium perfringens* and *Yersinia entercolitica* to be of concern.

Process of Identifying Pathogens of Concern

The fact that different agencies list different pathogens as being of concern to aging populations raises the question: How are pathogens of concern identified? Gendel explained that epidemiological and surveillance data, such as data from CDC FoodNet,[2] are the most useful type of data for determining whether a particular foodborne pathogen is more likely to infect or cause more serious illness in older adults. CDC FoodNet is a monitoring system that collects data at sites across the United States. The system covers about 15 percent of the U.S. population, providing a good estimate of total disease burden. Gendel then described several examples of how surveillance data are used to identify pathogens of concern, emphasizing again the importance of distinguishing between susceptibility versus severity of infection:

- *Listeria:* Again, all four agencies that Gendel examined list *Listeria monocytogenes* as being of concern to aging populations. CDC FoodNet data show that *Listeria* infection incidence rates are much higher in aging populations than younger ones. For both females and males, rates dramatically increase after middle age (i.e., at age 50–59). Data from Australia's OzFoodNet show the same trend of an increased incidence rate at about age 50–59. Similarly, in Canada, data from two different monitoring systems show that incidence rates increase dramatically with age (Clark et al., 2010). In addition to older adults being more susceptible to infection, older adults also experience more severe consequences of infection. Data collected for non-pregnancy associated *Listeria* severity in England and Wales from 1990–2007 show that the percentage of fatal cases increases with age, from about 10 percent in the 0–9 age group to about 45

[2] CDC FoodNet is the CDC's Foodborne Diseases Active Surveillance Network. Detailed information about its monitoring activities is available online at http://www.cdc.gov/FoodNet/.

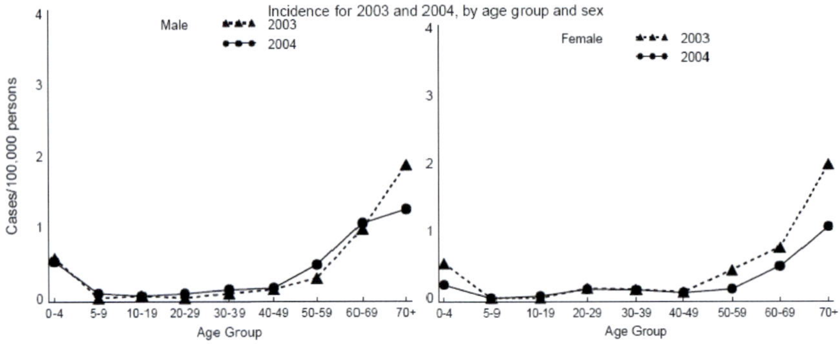

(a)

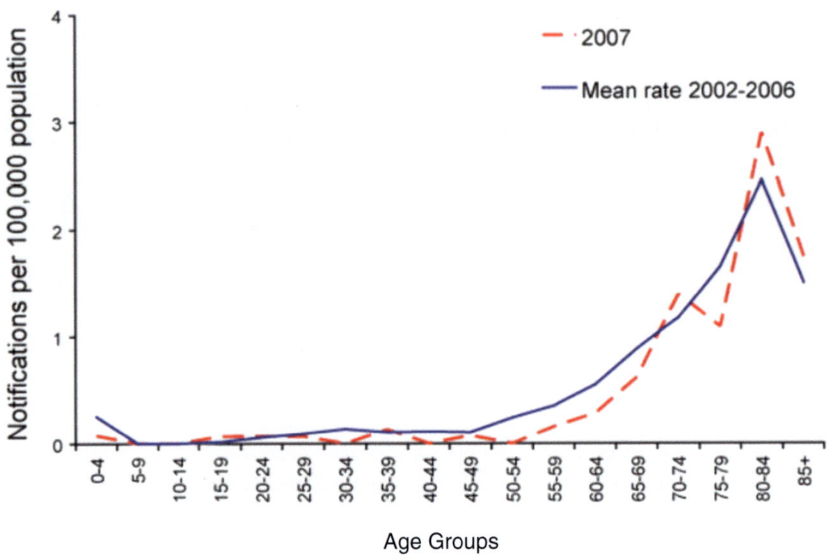

(b)

FIGURE 4-1 *Listeria* infection rates and the severity of illness from *Listeria* infection both increase with aging. Panels a, b, and c provide evidence of the increased incidence of *Listeria* infection with population age in the U.S. (a), Australia (b), and Canada (c). Panel (d) provides evidence of the increased severity (in terms of fatalities) of *Listeria* infection in England and Wales.
SOURCES: FoodNet Surveillance Report, 2004; OzFoodNet Australia, 2007; UK Advisory Committee on Microbiological Safety of Food, 2009; Clark et al., 2010.

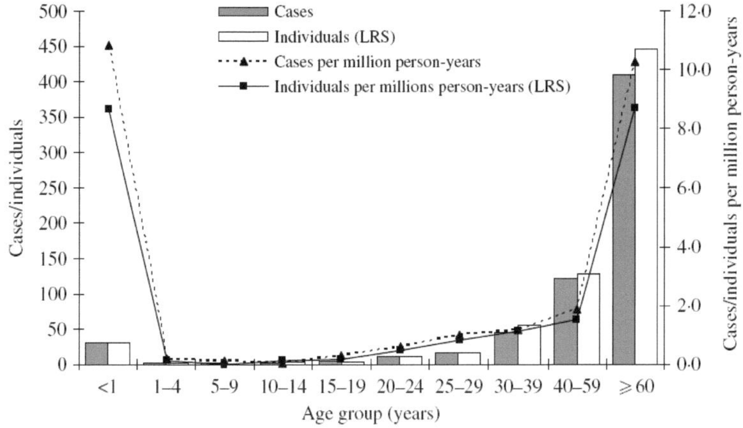

(c)

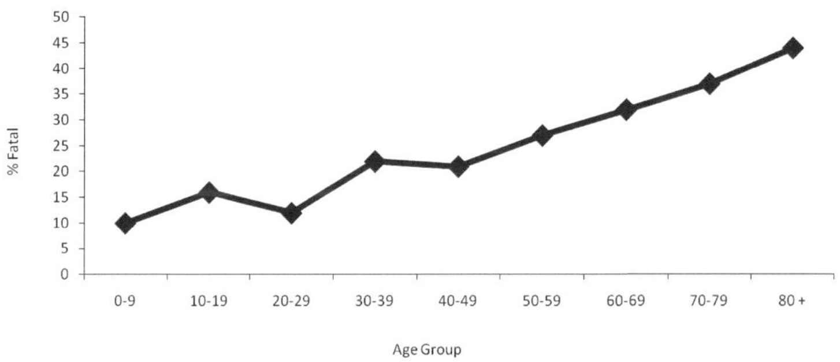

(d)

percent in the 80-and-over age group.[3] See Figure 4-1 for a summary of data on *Listeria* trends with aging.

- *Campylobacteria:* In contrast to *Listeria*, *Campylobacteria* data from CDC FoodNet show a much higher incidence in the very young and then, with aging, a decreasing and eventually constant rate. In other words, incidence does not increase with aging. Data from Australia's OzFoodNet demonstrates the same trend. While *Campylobacteria* is of interest since it is an extremely common foodborne illness, it is not necessarily any more common in older adults than it is in younger populations. Indeed, none of the four agencies that Gendel

[3] Available online: http://acmsf.food.gov.uk/acmsfreps/ (accessed July 28, 2010).

examined lists it as being of particular concern to aging populations. He remarked that the difference in incidence rates between *Listeria* and *Campylobacteria* is an example of how increased susceptibility to foodborne infectious disease with aging is not a general trend.

- *Shigella:* Data on *Shigella* incidence are not as clear-cut as with *Listeria* and *Campylobacteria*. Neither CDC FoodNet nor OzFoodNet show an increased incidence with age. Gendel speculated that when advisories are released warning older adults to avoid foods that may be contaminated with *Shigella*, it may be that older populations are not necessarily more susceptible to infection but are more susceptible to severe consequences of infection (e.g., diarrhea, vomiting).
- *Vibrio:* CDC FoodNet data show that *Vibrio* incidence rates by age differ between males and females, with incidence rates in males increasing dramatically with age. This is particularly true of *Vibrio vulnificus*. While this could indicate that males are more susceptible as they age, in fact susceptibility to *Vibrio* is affected by several kinds of underlying behavioral and medical conditions. It more likely reflects that fact that men are at a greater risk not because they are men, because they consume more shellfish as well as alcohol, and certain kinds of alcoholic conditions are underlying risk factors for *Vibrio* infection. The trend in *Vibrio* incidence is a good example of a trend that is confounded by other risk factors (i.e., eating shellfish).
- *Salmonella:* As with *Shigella*, CDC FoodNet data provide no clear indication that susceptibility to *Salmonella* infection increases with age. However, when outbreak data are examined more closely, it is clear that though incidence rates do not increase with age, severity of illness does. The percentage of people infected with *Salmonella* who then develop bacteremia increases dramatically with age (Blaser and Feldman, 1981). Likewise, the percentage of people infected with *Salmonella* that develop bacteriuria increases with age, particularly for females (Sivapalasingam et al., 2004).
- *E. coli* O157:H7: As with *Salmonella*, while CDC FoodNet data show low and constant levels of infection with aging, outbreak data from Scotland and China show that the percentage of cases with severe complications increases with age (Dundas et al., 2001; Zhu et al., 2009).

Gendel noted viral gastroenteritis and the lack of concern expressed by any of the four authorities about viruses as age-related problems, with the exception of norovirus. Norovirus is likely to cause diarrhea in older adults, thus the issue is probably that the consequences of the symptoms are what is more severe in older populations, rather than the incidence of disease.

Conclusion

In conclusion, Gendel claimed that susceptibility to foodborne pathogens in aging populations differs among microbes and is not just a matter of the immune system becoming dysfunctional as people age [which Meydani had argued in the previous session]. As he said, "Something about the pathogens themselves and the way that they interact with the body differs for different [pathogens]." Moreover, for many pathogens, the increased probability of severe outcomes is of greater concern than increased susceptibility to infection *per se*. Sometimes incidence rates increase with aging, sometimes incidence rates remain constant with aging but severity increases, and sometimes both incidence and severity increase with aging. Thus, Glendel suggested the problem is more nuanced than it might seem if one considers only changes in immune system function and general health characteristics.

CONTAMINANTS OF CONCERN

Presenter: Bernadene Magnuson

Magnuson began by noting the scarcity of data and information available on the effect of dietary contaminants on health during aging. Most of the evidence for the impact of contaminants in aging populations is for non-dietary contaminants, with many of the known associations coming from occupational exposures (e.g., to pesticides); and because occupational exposure is generally greater than dietary exposure, it is difficult to make inferences.

Magnuson identified three ways that exposure (i.e., including non-dietary exposure) to contaminants could play a role during aging:

- *Contaminants could promote aging by accelerating degenerative processes.* Examples include the association between increased exposure to cigarette smoking and the development of wrinkles (i.e., people who smoke develop more wrinkles), with considerable information available on the actual molecular mechanism for how this occurs; the known association between cognitive decline and the toxic effects of several heavy metals; hypothesized but debated associations between exposure to pesticides, heavy metals, and polychlorinated biphenyls (PCBs) and an increased risk of Parkinson's disease (i.e., some epidemiological reports support this hypothesis, others do not); and a clear association between contaminants or toxins that inhibit calcium absorption and bone integrity. Again, most of these data are from occupational, not dietary, exposure levels (Cummings, 2007; Bernhard and Laufer, 2008; Peterson et al., 2008). No clear relationships have been established for dietary levels of contaminants and these various degenerative processes.

- *Contaminants could accumulate over time and have adverse effects with advancing age, impacting the overall health status of the aging population.* Examples include heavy metals that accumulate in various organs, such as lead in bones, mercury in the brain, and cadmium in the kidney; and organochlorines, such as dichlorodiphenyltrichloroethane (DDT), PCBs, and chlordane that accumulate in adipose tissue. While lead toxicity is usually associated with neurological effects, a recent prospective study on bone lead concentrations and health outcomes in 868 men found that the strongest association was between the accumulation of bone lead and both all-cause and cardiovascular disease mortality (Weisskopf et al., 2009).
- *Older adults could be more vulnerable or susceptible to the adverse effects of toxic insult*, because of the way body composition changes with aging (i.e., aging is usually associated with a loss of lean muscle mass and increased adipose tissue), impaired cell and tissue function, and altered nutritional status (Ginsberg et al., 2005). Various specific factors play a role in this increased sensitivity with aging, including changes in liver physiology and function, changes in gastrointestinal (GI) function, changes in dietary patterns, increased use of dietary supplements, and increased potential for interactions between supplements and drugs.

With respect to changes in liver function, hepatic metabolic capacity decreases with advancing age, such that clearance (ability of the body to eliminate drugs) decreases and retention (half-life of drugs) increases. Drugs (or contaminants) remain at active levels for a longer time. Also, because of the increase in body fat percentage among older adults, lipophilic clearance decreases as well; and proteinuria results in a decreased plasma protein binding capacity. Both of these changes further impact the ability of the body to eliminate drugs and contaminants.

With respect to GI function, Magnuson noted that, as had been discussed in previous presentations, the function throughout the small and large intestines change little with age. Yet, studies on exposure to toxic substances conducted by her lab and others show that some changes that influence susceptibility to toxins do occur with aging. For example, she and her colleagues have demonstrated a loss of epidermal growth factor receptor-related protein function in an aged colon, which in turn increases the risk of colon cancer (Schmelz et al., 2004). The proteins offer protection against various toxins, and loss of function increases exposure to potential food carcinogens (e.g., those found in cooked meats). Magnuson's group has observed dramatic changes in the morphology of the aging colon of rats, with much less structure and fewer epithelial cells, which are likely responsible for changes in function and biological response to acute insult (Kwon and Magnuson, 2007, 2009).

Finally, changes in nutritional status, such as those caused by poor oral health or a loss of taste or smell, can affect susceptibility (Soliman et al., 1999; Hickson, 2006).

Assessing the Safety of Active Ingredients in Dietary Supplements

For the remainder of her talk, Magnuson discussed the widespread use of dietary supplements, the scarcity of safety data on the active ingredients in many dietary supplements, and the potential risks of dietary supplement-drug interactions.

Over 80 percent of Americans have tried at least one of the some 29,000 supplements on the market, and at least 40 percent of older Americans regularly use some form of herbal or specialty supplement. People, particularly the elderly, try or use supplements for various reasons: maintenance of overall health (most older adults no longer feel quite as invulnerable as they did at the age of 20 and start feeling a sense of their own mortality); increased energy (e.g., as reflected in the proliferation of energy drinks in the marketplace); memory improvement; prevention or treatment of illness; and slowing of the aging process.

Importantly, safety of the active ingredients of many dietary supplements is not tested to nearly the same extent that safety of food ingredients is tested. For example, there is no required testing for differences in susceptibility in older populations. In fact, usually the concern is with pregnant women, children, and infants. Unless there are other subpopulations that are of specific concern, everybody tends to get lumped together for risk assessment purposes. The lack of safety data is of concern given that dietary supplements have been contaminated in the past with heavy metals (lead, mercury, arsenic), organic solvents, pesticide residues, and other substances (e.g., melamine). Magnuson stated that some of these contaminants are "expected" (e.g., lead and mercury), but others like melamine "totally come out of the blue" and have never been considered potential contaminants. Even when recommended maximum levels for specific contaminants exist, those specifications are rarely enforced, leaving consumers little choice but to trust the reputation of the manufacturer. The challenge is even greater for products being imported from countries where quality control ranges from limited to non-existent. For example, a survey of herbal medicines imported from South Asia showed that 20 percent contained heavy metals in large enough quantities such that if a person were to take the recommended amount of oral supplement, he or she would be exceeding the recommended intake levels (of heavy metal) just from intake of the supplement alone (Saper et al., 2004).

In addition to the risk of contamination, older adults are also at greater risk of dietary supplement-drug interactions because of aging-related decreased metabolic capacity, increased likelihood of liver or kidney disease, and decreased capacity for tissue defense and repair. In a recent survey of older adults on the U.S.-Mexico border, 72.3 percent of adults surveyed reported using multiple medications, including 38.5 percent who took five or more; 16.2 percent reported taking multiple herbs; 26 percent multiple supplements; and 9 percent multiple nutraceuticals (Loya et al., 2009). Forty-six percent of adults surveyed were identified as being at risk for a drug-drug interaction, and 32 percent were identified as being at high risk for a drug-herbal product interaction (Loya et al., 2009).

The problem, Magnuson explained, is that there is not much known about these drug-herbal product interactions, given there are approximately 29,000 herbal products on the market and most of the information collected is based on case reports. Many people do not admit they are taking dietary supplements, unless the supplement becomes popular, as Goji berry juice did in Canada in 2008.

Magnuson's laboratory has been investigating the issue of age-related changes in drug/toxin-supplement interactions. In particular, they are interested in age-related differences in the efficacy of two dietary supplements commonly used as a form of chemoprotection against cancer: curcumin and soy isoflavones.

- Curcumin is believed to have antioxidant, anti-inflammatory, anti-aging, and anti-cancer (against many forms of cancer) properties. While its chemopreventive capacity is well documented in young animals, Magnuson's team sought to explore its chemopreventive capacity in older animals by feeding differently aged rats diets supplemented with curcumin (Kwon et al., 2004). Because it is an antioxidant, they expected that the supplement would become even more chemopreventive with aging. However, they found that while curcumin reduced early neoplastic lesions in both young (6 weeks old) and old rats (about 2 years), it had no effect in mature rats (1 year). This unexpected finding was subsequently shown to be likely a result of age-related differences in induction of apoptosis (Kwon and Magnuson, 2009).
- Soy isoflavones are believed to prevent cancer (breast and prostate) and provide relief from post-menopausal symptoms. In another study, Magnuson's team fed diets supplemented with soy isoflavones to differently aged female rats (Daly et al., 2007). One week

after starting the experimental diet, the rats were treated with a colon carcinogen. They expected that older rats would be less sensitive or responsive because of lower rates of absorption as well as lower estrogen and estrogen receptor levels. However, shockingly, they found immediate evidence of age-related toxicity, with old rats (22 months) rapidly becoming very ill. Half of the rats in the old age group died within the first 96 hours. The young rats showed no signs of toxicity. The soy isoflavone diet had no benefit for any age rat in terms of inhibiting the development of colon cancer lesions. Additionally, older rats that were fed the supplemented diet lost significantly more weight during the course of the experiment than older rats fed the control diet. The soy isoflavone supplement had no effect on weight in younger rats. Also, older rats fed the supplemented diet showed a dramatic increase in serum estradiol with aging, even though older rats were consuming less soy isoflavone per body weight than younger rats were (serum estradiol levels normally decrease with aging, as was the case with rats fed the control diet).

In sum, dietary curcumin was not chemoprotective in mature animals, although it did reduce colon cancer lesions in young and old rats, demonstrating age-dependent mechanisms. Soy isoflavone supplementation also resulted in very different responses among three age groups of rats, with older female rats becoming very ill, suggesting that soy isoflavones augment or trigger age-related toxicity. The soy isoflavone study raises the question: Why? Is this a drug-diet interaction? Because supplementation with soy isoflavones affected estrogen and estrogen-responsive tissues in older rats, might it have adverse effects with other hormone-dependent cancers? Magnuson stated that the adverse effects of soy isoflavones in aged female animals observed in their pilot study needs further examination, because older women are the primary target population for the consumption of soy supplements.

Conclusion

In conclusion, Magnuson reiterated that there is very little information available on the effect of dietary contaminants on health during aging, but that changes in diet and physiology during aging clearly increase the risk for adverse effects. Dietary supplements are an important source of contaminants, given the widespread use of supplements among older adults and the prevalence of contamination in supplements. The high use of both supplements and drugs in older adults also increases the likelihood of supplement-drug interactions. Lack of awareness around patient use of supplements in older adults makes it difficult to monitor and gather information on possible interactions, and what is known about interactions in the young cannot be used to predict effects in older adults.

PROCESSING AND FORMULATION ADVANCES TO DECREASE FOOD SAFETY RISKS

Presenter: Michael Doyle

Doyle began by posing the question: What has the industry done and what can be done to develop products that are safe for aging populations? He shared a list of foods of concern, which was almost identical to the list that Sundlof had shown in an earlier session: sprouts (e.g., alfalfa, broccoli), raw meat and poultry, raw fish and seafood, raw milk and milk dairy products, fresh fruits and vegetables, unpasteurized fruit juices, deli meats, frankfurters, and cold smoked seafoods. Foodborne illnesses in aging populations, Doyle observed, are largely associated with consumption of raw and uncooked foods.

The industry has developed several different types of interventions and continues to develop new ways to ensure food safety. Doyle identified four categories of interventions:

- Physical (e.g., heat, ionizing radiation, high pressure, ultraviolet [UV] light)
- Gas (e.g., modified atmospheres)
- Biological (e.g., bacteriophage, competitive exclusion bacteria)
- Chemical (e.g., organic acids, oxidizing agents, bacteriocins)

Thermal processing technologies can be the "easiest" to apply and are the most traditional technologies used to ensure the safety of foods. Steam and hot water approaches have been used for decades for pasteurization and commercial sterilization, and there are also some newer innovative microwave and ohmic heating (liquids/pumpable) technologies. The problem with heat is that although the end result is a safe food, it has a cooked flavor, which Doyle explained is not always considered a desirable quality. Some of the non-thermal physical processing technologies and chemical treatments provide ways around this problem with end products that are not only safe but also taste and look fresh. For the remainder of his talk, Doyle discussed these non-thermal physical and chemical ways of protecting foods from pathogen contamination, their advantages and disadvantages, and their actual and potential applications.

Non-Thermal Physical Processing Technologies

Non-thermal physical processes are those that do not require high temperatures and which therefore can have several advantages from both a taste and nutrition perspective. Not only do non-thermally processed foods not taste cooked, if given a sporicidal treatment, they may not require the addition of preservatives which means that the sodium content could be kept low. Doyle highlighted several types of non-thermal processing technologies.

High Hydrostatic Pressure

Many companies utilize this type of technology, which involves applying high-pressure water (e.g., 87,000 pounds per square inch [psi]) to foods. The high pressure precludes the need for high temperatures. Foods can be subject to pressures between 100 and 800 megapascal (MPa) and can be treated at temperatures from 0°C to above 100°C. Exposure times range from a few seconds to more than 20 minutes. This technology works best on moist foods that can withstand high-pressure water without being crushed, such as liquids, pastes, and meats. For example, it does not work very well on lettuce but does work well on apple juice.

High hydrostatic pressure technology has several benefits: foods retain their nutritional, flavor, and color characteristics; the process kills vegetative cells of many different pathogens (e.g., *Salmonella*, *Listeria monocytogenes*); it works for both liquid and solid foods and with or without packaging; it uniformly kills microbes regardless of size, shape, and food composition; and it precludes the need for preservatives, which in turn can reduce sodium content. But it also has its drawbacks: it is not a continuous system (i.e., it is batch or semi-continuous) and therefore cannot be used for beverages that are made on a continuous basis; it does not kill spores reliably at temperatures below about 90°C; and it is more expensive than canning or freezing.

Commercial applications include apple juice and other fruit juices, smoothies, deli meats, guacamole, oysters, and clams. With oysters and clams, not only does high hydrostatic pressure kill *Vibrio* without killing the shell organism, it also has added value because of the fact that it enables easier shucking of the shell.

Ionizing Radiation

While ionizing radiation, or irradiation, technology is approved for many uses (i.e., spices, fruits, vegetables, wheat, flour, pork, chicken, red meats, shell eggs, seeds for sprouts, mollusks, lettuce, spinach, and food for the U.S. space program), few products on the market today are protected through it. Doyle argued that ionizing radiation has greater potential and more applications than are currently being realized and there may be niche market opportunities, for example the production of irradiated foods for aging populations at high risk of acquiring severe foodborne illnesses.

There are several benefits of ionizing radiation: it kills pathogens, preserves food, and disinfects; and 50 years of testing and safety studies have deemed it safe when used at dosages that would pasteurize food. But there are also significant drawbacks: its lack of consumer acceptance; it is generally not useful for destroying viruses, toxins, and prions; and it may produce off odors and off flavors in foods (e.g., some people describe it as producing a "wet dog" odor). With respect to consumer acceptance, Doyle mentioned irradiated ground beef and how, after being marketed nationwide but not selling well, irradiated ground beef was taken off the market and the company responsible went bankrupt.

There are several different types of ionizing radiation technologies:

- *Gamma irradiation* involves the use of radionucleotides (Cobalt 60, Cesium 137, or other photons) as the ionization energy source, whereby the radionucleotides are simply exposed to the food. Unlike the other ionizing radiation technologies, the radionucleotides are always present in the processing plant.
- *Electron beam processing* involves focusing a beam of electrons onto the food. Unlike gamma irradiation, electron beam processes can be turned on and off and are therefore not always present in the plant. The downside is the technology has a very low penetration and only works for relatively thin layers of food.
- *X-ray processing* involves using electrons that have been converted into X-rays. Like an electron beam, X-rays can be turned on and off. They also have a high penetration and can therefore be used for thicker foods.

Listeristatic/listericidal Additives for the Mitigation of Listeria Monocytogenes *Contamination of Ready-to-Eat Meat Products*

Doyle noted that as Gendel had already discussed, the severity of illness from *Listeria* infection increases with advancing age, so it is an important threat to consider when formulating new food safety interventions. Ready-to-eat meat products are subject to *Listeria* contamination primarily during the slicing and packaging process after the meat has been cooked. *Listeria* can persist and grow at refrigeration temperatures, and most luncheon meats have a refrigeration shelf life of about one to two months. The food industry has developed several different commercial treatments for the prevention of later *Listeria* growth at refrigeration temperature, including heat (i.e., submersion of packaged meat into 90˚C water for two minutes, which does not cook the inside meat but does slightly cook the outside meat, which is where *Listeria* usually grows); high hydrostatic pressure processing (only a few companies are using this technology); and chemical antimicrobials, namely the combined use of potassium lactate and sodium diacetate.

Doyle described a study showing how growth of *Listeria* in untreated vacuum-packed, sliced, cooked ham increases tremendously over time (from 0 to 40 days at 4˚C), while there is no growth at all in meat treated with a solution of 2.5 percent sodium lactate and 0.25 percent sodium acetate (Blom et al., 1997) (Figure 4-2). When the same product is slightly temperature abused (i.e., stored at 9˚C instead of 4˚C), the chemical treatment no longer totally suppresses growth, although growth is not nearly as rapid as it is without treatment. Taken together, these results suggest that chemical treatment is both time and temperature dependent. The longer the storage

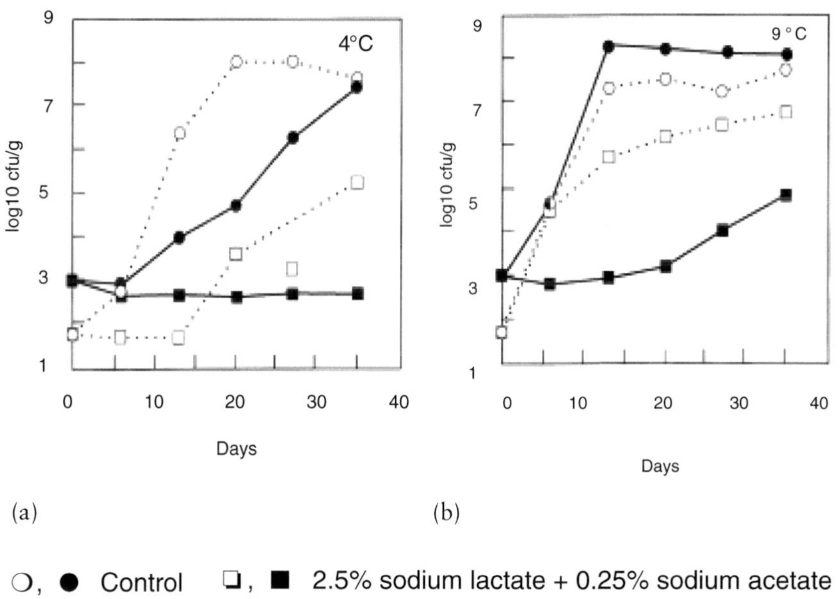

FIGURE 4-2 Growth of *Listeria monocytogenes* (closed symbols) and lactic acid bacteria (open symbols) in vacuum-packed, sliced, cooked ham stored at two different temperatures: (a) at 4°C and (b) at 9°C, with or without treatment with sodium lactate and sodium acetate.
SOURCE: Blom et al., 1997.

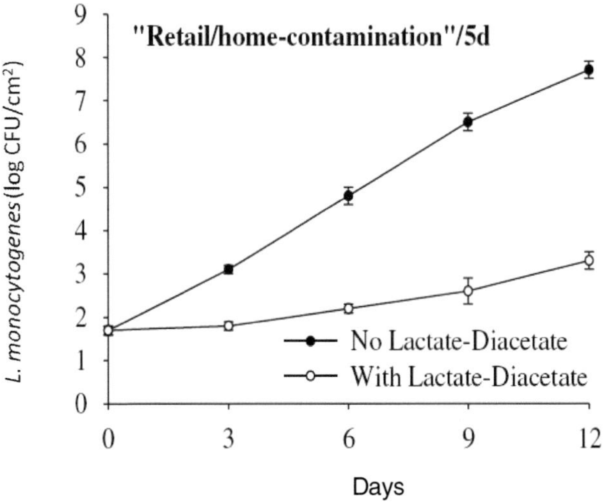

FIGURE 4-3 Growth of *Listeria monocytogenes* in uncured turkey breast meat stored at 7°C for 12 days, with and without added lactate-diacetate.
SOURCE: Lianou et al., 2007.

time and the warmer the temperature, the less likely it is that growth will be suppressed.

In another study, with vacuum-packaged uncured turkey breast meat stored at 7°C for up to 12 days, again the chemical treatment (in this case 1.5 percent sodium lactate and 0.05 percent sodium diacetate) suppressed *Listeria* growth (Lianou et al., 2007). In the untreated package, the *Listeria* population increased from about 100 cells at day 0 to 10^8 cells at day 12 (Figure 4-3).

Doyle stated that because lactate-diacetate provides such a high level of public health protection by mitigating the growth of *Listeria monocytogenes* on high-risk deli meats during in-home and retail use, it is widely used by the food industry today.

Antimicrobial Washes for Fresh Produce and Poultry

Doyle explained how he and his colleagues recently discovered that the use of levulinic acid in combination with a detergent, sodium dodecyl sulfate (SDS), is a highly effective way to kill harmful bacteria on produce and poultry (Zhao et al., 2009). They showed that neither chemical on its own suppresses either *Salmonella* or *E. coli* O157:H7 growth on lettuce with exposure times of 5 minutes or less, but that, together, the combination "is like dynamite." Treatment with a 0.5 percent levulinic acid and 0.05 percent SDS solution results in a dramatic reduction in *Salmonella* or *E. coli* O157:H7 contamination after just five minutes of exposure. Treatment with a 3 percent levulinic acid and 1 percent SDS solution results in complete reduction of all detectable microbes within just one minute. The beauty of this technique, Doyle said, is that levulinic acid does not destroy the integrity of the food being treated, as is the case with lactic acid and other organic acids, which usually cause lettuce leaves (or leafy greens) to turn brown and wilt within a couple days of exposure. As part of the same study, the researchers also found that treatment with 3 percent levulinic acid plus 2 percent SDS killed all detectable *Salmonella* on poultry wings within two minutes of exposure.

Doyle commented on the many advantages of a levulinic acid plus SDS antimicrobial treatment:

- Studies have shown that, depending on concentrations and exposure time, the chemical combination has strong antimicrobial activity not just against *Salmonella* and *E. coli* O157:H7 but also *Listeria monocytogenes*, *Yersinia pestis*, *Bacillus anthracis*, and *Norovirus*.
- Its antimicrobial activity is not inactivated by the organic load, which is what happens with chlorine (if there is blood or soil in the tanks used to wash poultry, it will inactivate the chlorine).
- It is non-corrosive to stainless steel and non-irritating to skin.
- It removes biofilms.
- It is fast-acting.
- Foods can retain their sensory properties (color, appearance, texture, odor).

Reducing Portion Size

In addition to all of these various existing and innovative technologies aimed at protecting against or suppressing microbial growth in foods, many companies have also begun reducing the portion sizes of products in packages. Doyle remarked that this is commendable, given the additional cost of producing these that may not be fully recovered. Hot dogs, for example, are now available in packages of five and not just packages of 10. Many older adults are not likely to go through 10 hot dogs, or even five, in just one sitting. This is an important food safety preventative measure, given that opening a package and then putting the unused resealed hot dogs back in the refrigerator creates the potential for *Listeria* contamination and growth.

Conclusion

In conclusion, Doyle emphasized the market sustainability of three processes in particular:

- high hydrostatic pressure processing of deli meats, fruit juices, and oysters;
- the formulation of ready-to-eat meats with listeriostatic chemicals (i.e., potassium lactate and sodium diacetate); and
- the packaging of smaller portion sizes.

Challenges to applying some of the other new processing technologies and formulations to mitigate pathogen contamination of foods are largely related to sensory changes (e.g., changes in smell or taste), added costs, and consumer acceptance or willingness to pay more for foods that have been processed or formulated using these technologies. However, perhaps with a growing population of older adults, a niche of sufficient market size will eventually develop such that production of new lines of "pathogen-free" foods created from some of these other technologies (e.g., irradiation) can be sustainable.

PACKAGING AND STORAGE CHALLENGES AND SOLUTIONS TO DECREASING SAFETY RISKS

Presenter: Aaron Brody

Brody remarked that the goal of his talk would be to describe the key role played by the packaging industry in meeting consumer food and nutrition needs and desires. He stated that the industry is doing this better than it has at any other time in history and at a lower cost and with less environmental impact. Packaging costs fewer than 7 percent of the retail price of food, which itself is at its lowest cost in history; food expenses today amount to fewer than 11 percent of disposable income, even with away-from-home eating.

What Is Packaging?

Brody defined packaging as the separation of a product from the environment. He stated that a package is not merely a piece of material or a structure; it is a holistic system, with its primary purpose being protection "against an always hostile natural environment." Without packaging, industrialized society would not exist. Not only does packaging enable the delivery of goods from one place to another, it also enables eating. About 60 percent of all packaging is food packaging.

One of the primary functions of food packaging is protection from the natural environment. Food packaging protects against oxygen, moisture, water, microorganisms, light, dirt, odors, animals, and humans; and without food packaging, food waste would be over 50 percent. Food packaging also allows for delivery to its intended recipient(s); protects foods during distribution (e.g., from the impact, vibration, and compression that occurs during transit); retains the nutritional quality and sensory characteristics of the initial product; allows for an extended commercial shelf life; communicates information; allows for accessing and dispensing of contents (e.g., Brody mentioned the development of easy-open soup packages that eliminate the need for can opener); and serves other functions. Industry "guidelines" for packaging include safety, protection of the contents, consumer convenience (ease of access and use), facilitation of finding products, attractiveness to a diverse customer base, applicability for away-from-home eating (which amounts to about half of all food consumption), and minimal environmental impact.

Recent Developments and Innovations in Food Packaging

Brody discussed several recent developments in food packaging, emphasizing that the weight of packaging per unit food is at its lowest in history. The use of heavier-weight glass, metal, and high-caliper paperboard structures is declining, while the use of lightweight plastic and other flexible structures is growing. He showed several pictures of the wide variety of new types of food packaging systems currently being marketed, and he reiterated the important role of packaging in ensuring microbiological safety.

Plastics and Other Flexible Structures

Carbonated beverages were the first beverage or food to be packaged in lightweight, non-breakable polyester bottles instead of glass (in 1977). Today, many different beverages and foods are packaged in plastic bottles, including fruit beverages, jams, tomato sauce, and even beer. For example, instead of all-steel cans, roasted and ground coffee is now being packaged in lighter-weight, more unitizing (larger quantities can be moved at once) plastic containers; and hot-fill high acid fluid foods (e.g., tomato paste) are being packaged in laminated flexible pouches instead of metal cans. Plastics are also being used to design other types of packages, like microwavable, individual unit portion, and liner-less composite paperboard packages. Brody explained that no single plastic material is "magic" and that different materials are often used in combination.

Aseptic Packaging

Another recent development is aseptic packaging, which involves sterilizing the product and package separately and then assembling them together in a sterile environment. This reduces the amount of heat used on the product, thereby extending its shelf life, while simultaneously allowing for the use of just about any packaging material (e.g., composite paperboard bricks, barrier plastic cups, lightweight packaging). The use of very carefully temperature-controlled distribution systems extends shelf life even further.

Gas-Permeable Packaging

Another recent trend is the use of gas-permeable packaging for fresh-cut vegetables. By giving the vegetables a little bit of oxygen, their shelf life lasts longer (i.e., two weeks in a refrigerated environment).

Packaging for Consumer Delight or Convenience

The industry is seeking new ways to "delight" customers, for example by using differently shaped cans (instead of cylindrical cans), as well as new ways to make products more convenient. Examples of new convenience foods include "no drain" tuna, which is packaged in a reduced liquid retort pouches instead of heavy metal cans, and ready-to-eat fruit bowls.

Conclusion

Brody ended by summarizing current and future trends in food packaging. He mentioned increased use of flexible packaging, which reduces both the product weight and the risk of breakage that would exist if glass were used. He showed products shaped for convenience and portability, such as single-serving packages and heat-and-eat packages, where the package serves as the processing aid and the serving container. He also mentioned that some packaging methods require less heat for sterilization, which boosts the nutritional value of the products, making these types of packaging potentially attractive for new product development.

PANEL DISCUSSION ON IMPLICATIONS FOR REGULATORS, EDUCATORS, AND THE FOOD INDUSTRY

A panel discussion followed the four presentations. David J. Greenblatt of Tufts University School of Medicine, Boston, Massachusetts, was invited to join the four speakers on stage and provide initial comments.

Interactions Between Nutrients and Prescription Medications

Presenter: David Greenblatt

To begin the panel discussion, Greenblatt offered some brief thoughts on the interaction between nutrients and prescription medications. He noted that pharmaceuticals have advanced at an incredible pace over the past 20 to 30 years and that one reason the U.S. population is aging so successfully is because of these and other biomedical advances. He said that when talking about the aging population and nutrition, one is automatically talking about people on medication. This raises questions about whether and how medications interact with nutrients. The "prototype" of a nutrient-drug interaction, he said, is "the grapefruit juice story."

In the early 1990s, pharmacology researcher David Bailey and his team at the University of Western Ontario were the first to report an interaction between grapefruit juice and the calcium channel antagonist felodipine (Edgar et al., 1992). They reported that felodipine in combination with grapefruit juice caused about a five to tenfold increase in plasma felodipine concentration, resulting in adverse effects in many individuals. Knowledge of these adverse effects eventually led to hundreds of scientific studies but also a tremendous amount of inaccurate press and widespread public belief that it was not safe to drink grapefruit juice with any medication. Through a combined effort on the part of both the biomedical and nutritional science communities, researchers eventually learned that the interaction revolved around the enzyme cytochrome P450-3A (CYP3A).

Greenblatt explained that CYP3A intervenes at two points in the drug metabolism process. With an oral dose of the drug, the drug first passes through the mucosa of the small bowel, which Greenblatt described as containing substantial quantities of CYP3A. There, any drugs that are substrates for metabolism by CYP3A maybe metabolized. Whatever drug remains (i.e., has not been metabolized) enters the portal circulation and the liver, where there is more CYP3A, before entering the systemic circulation. Again, in the liver, there is another opportunity for metabolism. So there are two opportunities for first-pass metabolism (i.e., pre-systematic extraction). Since grapefruit juice contains furanocoumarins, which interact with CYP3A in the small bowel, individuals who drink grapefruit juice may be less able to metabolize drugs that serve as substrates for CYP3A in the small bowel, and they may end up with greater amounts of drug in systemic circulation.

Greenblatt emphasized that only a few drugs are of concern and that the interaction is a product only of grapefruit juice, no other fruit product. Only buspirone, felodipine and simvastatin have shown probable interactions (e.g., see Lilja et al., 1998), and only a handful of additional drugs having shown possible interactions (triazolam, midazolam, diazepam, nisoldipine, lovastatin, carbamazepine, cyclosporine) (Greenblatt, 2010). His advice to patients already taking any of these drugs with grapefruit juice and not showing any signs of an adverse effect is to continue what they are doing, as presumably their dose has been adjusted to achieve the proper pharmacologic and clinical effects. However, for patients who are taking any of the three drugs that have shown probable interaction, he advised that grapefruit juice be avoided. With the other drugs that have shown possible interactions, he would advise caution but would not necessarily advise avoiding grapefruit juice. Although pomegranate, cranberry, grape, lime, pomelo, and tangerine juices have all shown interactions with CYP3A in a test tube, the interaction is reversible. With grapefruit juice, the interaction is irreversible: the only way to increase the level of active enzyme is to produce more. This is a property only of grapefruit juice; it does not apply to any other fruit products.

Lack of Funding for Nutrition Research

Greenblatt also commented on how both overall endowment values and annual rates of return on investments have fallen dramatically over the past several years, for "probably every university in the nation." He commented that financial reasons have created a "hugely reduced and less friendly" university environment for biomedical research, which coupled with a decrease in NIH funding over the last 5 to 10 years, stimulus money notwithstanding, raises serious questions about how some of these critical nutrition questions will be answered.

Panel Discussion

The four presentations and Greenblatt's remarks prompted many comments and questions from the audience about the evidence for nutrient-drug interactions in older adults, data on foodborne infectious diseases in older adults, the challenges of developing innovative packaging for older adults, the complexity of the issue of consumer acceptance (i.e., of food technologies), and the use of chlorine as a decontaminant.

Drug-Nutrient Interactions

The first remarks were directed toward Dr. Magnuson. An audience member commented that her soy isoflavone study in rats appeared to involve only 11 animals, then asked whether she or others had ever examined the impact of standard rat chow, which contains soy isolate, on longevity. First, Magnuson remarked that the data she presented were from a preliminary study. She explained that the study began with 7 animals in each of the three age/treatment groups and that the number in the end was as low because of unanticipated deaths that occurred in the study. Five of the 21 rats fed the soy supplement died before the end of the experiment while all animals on the control diet (n = 21) survived to term. The researchers had not anticipated age-related differences in toxicity. The dose of soy isoflavones they used was lower than the reported NOAEL (no-observable-adverse-effect level) of 120 mg/kg/day determined in a 28-day repeated dose study with genistein in male and female rats, well below doses of up to 500 mg/kg/day that have been used in previous chemoprevention studies. Then, she explained that the treatment involved adding soy isoflavone supplements to a standard AIN-96 diet and that the goal was to examine the effects of a supplemental level of soy isoflavone, not the effects of soy protein isolate.

Magnuson later clarified that she and her group chose to examine curcumin and soy isoflavones because of "the plethora of information on beneficial effects on those." Their data suggest, however, that there is insufficient information to be making those claims across all age groups. It is unclear why the nutrients have adverse effects in certain situations. She urged that more attention be paid to these types of very dramatic effects.

Later during the panel discussion, Greenblatt was asked if the grapefruit juice story he had told was the "last word" on drug-nutrient interactions. Greenblatt said that grapefruit juice is the "best" and "most dramatic" example. He argued that isolated case reports of interactions are useful for guiding future research but do not by themselves prove cause-and-effect; and that many animal studies may be irrelevant to human health because of enzymatic, hepatic blood flow, GI physiology, and other differences. Based on data from controlled human pharmacokinetic studies in which a drug was examined both before and after exposure to the nutrient in question, "there are precious few [examples] compared to grapefruit juice."

Incidence of Foodborne Infection and Severity of Illness in Older Adults

Gendel was asked why the incidence of some foodborne pathogens is higher in older adults and to what extent the data he discussed reflect the fact that someone with symptoms is more likely to seek help (and therefore be included in a surveillance data set) than someone who is infected but not showing symptoms. Gendel replied that the observed effects are real effects, given that FoodNet and other monitoring systems capture as much data as they do and make every effort to remove the medical intervention effect (i.e., whether somebody has sought medical treatment or not) from the system. For example, the Canadian *Listeria* data that he presented were obtained from two independent monitoring systems, and they both showed the same trend.

Packaging for Older Consumers

There were several remarks and questions regarding packaging. Brody was asked whether any of the packaging materials that he described have been tested to determine if any chemical residues might be leaching into food products. He responded that, yes, there have been many such studies. He commented on recent media headlines about bisphenol A (BPA), which is used primarily as a building block for the epoxy polymers in can liners. He said that FDA would be issuing a report on BPA very soon and that, in general, plastics are without question one of the most studied materials in world history with respect to chemical leaching. He said that while nobody can guarantee their absolute safety, evidence to date indicates that today's packaging materials are safe, especially when compared to what has been used in the past. Later during the discussion, there was another comment about BPA and the need to be very careful when measuring BPA, as BPA has been known to leach out of materials used (e.g., PEEK [polyether ether ketone] tubing) for BPA analytical procedures.

Another audience member commented that, while advances in packaging have made it easier to open certain products, "one of the ways that you are keeping elderly people safe from the food inside is that they still can't get to all of it." Often, the questioner said, older adults have difficulties opening some of the newer types of packaging, such as the fruit cups with pull-off lids, because of limited mobility in their fingers. This raises the question, how conscious is the packaging industry of the needs of older adults when designing new ways to package food products? Brody said that the industry shares an "extremely high level of consciousness" about the need to make products more accessible to older adults, as well as the need to keep children from opening packages that they should not be accessing. Brody mentioned ring-top pulls, peelable packaging, and slider zip loc bags as examples of the type of ongoing improvements being made with packaging. Many of these improvements are based on efficacy trials and other tests. However, with some 15,000 new packages introduced into the market every year, not every new package goes through the same testing procedures.

Another audience member mentioned a focus group study currently under way in Manitoba, Canada, with the goal of gaining a better understanding of how to design and develop food products for baby boomers.

While there has been improvement in packaging, some of the baby boomers participating in the study have been commenting on the difficulties with opening some of these new types of packages. For example, older adults with arthritis have reported difficulties opening the supposedly easy-open cans because they can't lift the lids with their fingers. So they use dull knives to open lids and, if that doesn't work, they'll bang cans on counters until the lids pop open. Or, they use scissors to try to pull lids open. Also, with many of the juices with antioxidant properties, the containers are very large and difficult to pour, again making them difficult to use. People who live alone end up not buying those products. So even with the introduction of new packaging, issues remain. Is the industry conducting any tests to determine how baby boomers and older adults open all of these new packages? Brody responded that yes, the industry is involved with focus group and other types of testing. He mentioned packaging industry trade magazines and journals as a source of information on the type of studies being conducted.

The Complexity of Consumer Acceptance

A comment that Doyle had made during his presentation about irradiated foods prompted an audience member to comment on the complexity of the issue of consumer acceptance. Consumer acceptance of risk depends on many factors, such as taste and cost. With respect to taste, irradiated beef reportedly tasted like wet dog to some consumers and singed hair to others. With respect to cost, irradiated beef was sold as safer and was therefore sold at a higher price in an attempt to recoup some of the cost, and most consumers probably did a fairly intuitive cost-benefit analysis and concluded that the higher cost was not worth reducing the risk of bacterial contamination. It is important to recognize this complexity and not draw the wrong conclusions. Some people have concluded that the failure of irradiated beef was a result of irresponsible propaganda, when in fact the situation was much more complicated than that. Consumers were making a "complicated, nuanced decision."

In response to these comments, Brody remarked that the unpleasant taste from irradiation occurs only when the official maximum dose is exceeded. Magnuson agreed with the audience member, stating that the remarks "hit on a very important point" about the complexity of public perception and consumer acceptance. For example, with dietary supplements, cost is not the issue for most consumers. Public perception is that because a supplement is "natural," it is therefore safe.

The Use of Active Chlorine as a Decontaminant

Doyle remarked that all new technologies come at a price and that the industry faces a tremendous challenge in terms of developing technologies that can be used to ensure safe food that still looks, smells, and tastes good. The challenge is especially difficult with those foods that are of greatest risk: fresh, uncooked foods. This remark prompted a question about the use of active chlorine to minimize *Salmonella* and *Camplyobacter* contamination in poultry products. The questioner noted that U.S. poultry plants use active chlorine for food decontamination purposes, but the European Commission does not allow the use of this practice in European plants. He asked the panelists their opinions on the use of a chemical that has toxic properties but that also effectively kills pathogens. The questioner also noted that there have been some claims that active chlorine is not efficacious at killing *Salmonella*. Doyle remarked that active chlorine is very effective at killing both *Campylobacter* and *Salmonella* "as long as the water is clear and clean." He reiterated that an organic load (e.g., blood, residue) in the chill water tanks or other liquids used to process poultry neutralizes active chlorine and makes it ineffective. Other factors, such as the hardness of the water used in the plant, also play a role. The U.S. industry uses active chlorine because it is relatively inexpensive compared with other disinfectants. There are other products that work better than active chlorine and that work well even in the presence of organic load, but they are more expensive. Companies often use these more expensive products when problems arise but then, when the problem is cleared, they revert to using active chlorine for routine decontamination. He noted that one of the alternatives is peracetic acid, which is not only more expensive than active chlorine but is also corrosive to equipment.

Campylobacter *Infection and Effects on Individuals of Different Ages*

The final query, directed to Gendel, was about the reason for the consistent incidence rate for *Campylobacter* infections. The audience member questioned whether older consumers' lack of increased susceptibility to infection, especially compared to the very young, is due to immunity that has built up throughout life. Gendel replied that there is no protective immunity against such pathogens, and said that perhaps children show a higher incidence of infection than older adults because they are more likely to get checked if something is wrong.

5

Nutrition Concerns for Aging Populations

Moderated by Johanna Dwyer of the National Institutes of Health (NIH) and the Jean Mayer U.S. Department of Agriculture (USDA) Human Nutrition Research Center on Aging (HNRCA) at Tufts University, Boston, Massachusetts, this session included four presentations. Katherine Tucker, also of the Jean Mayer USDA HNRCA at Tufts University, spoke about diet quality issues in aging populations. Stephen Barnes of the University of Alabama, Birmingham, discussed functional foods (i.e., foods with health benefits beyond what their traditional nutrients provide) and the challenge of bioavailability. He emphasized that not all functional foods, like soy, are necessarily alike with respect to their health-promoting benefits, depending on how they are processed. Luigi Fontana of Washington University, St. Louis, Missouri, and the Italian National Institute of Health, Rome, Italy, discussed recent research on caloric restriction and is effects on longevity and age-associated diseases. Both Fontana and Tucker also addressed the issue of protein intake in older adults. Finally, Jim Kirkwood of General Mills discussed the importance of combining science with consumer desires when considering how to formulate foods that older consumers will actually purchase and eat. He emphasized the importance of understanding "what really matters to consumers" when developing and marketing food products, a theme that was revisited at length in the session on communication (see Chapter 6). The session ended with a panel discussion.

DIET QUALITY ISSUES FOR AGING POPULATIONS

Presenter: Katherine Tucker

Tucker remarked that the focus of her talk would be on how dietary needs change with aging, which nutrients in particular are important for aging populations, and the challenge of achieving access to and consumption of a high quality diet given the obstacles already discussed by other speakers (e.g., loss of appetite, oral health decline, mobility constraints).

How Dietary Needs Change with Aging

Dietary needs change with aging in several ways:

- People become less active, their metabolism slows, their energy requirement decreases, all of which mean that they need to eat less.
- Recent research demonstrates that because older adults' abilities to absorb and utilize many nutrients become less efficient, their nutrient requirements (particularly as a function of body mass) actually increase. Tucker mentioned that the last set of nutrition recommendations issued by the Institute of Medicine (IOM) include separate recommendations for people age 70 and above for this reason (IOM, 2006).
- Tucker noted that as some of the previous speakers had discussed, chronic conditions and medications can affect nutrition requirements. For example, in addition to drug-nutrient interactions affecting drug metabolism, some drug-nutrient interactions are also nutrient wasting. This is especially true of the B vitamins.

Maintaining a nutrient-dense diet is critically important for older adults because of the impact of food intake on health. Years of research have demonstrated that diet quality has a huge effect on physical condition, cognitive condition, bone health, eye health, vascular function, and the immune system. Yet, this can be challenging to achieve for several reasons:

- As Pelchat discussed, aging is often accompanied by a loss of appetite and changes in taste and smell, all of which can lead to more limited food choices and lower intake of healthful foods.
- As Jensen discussed, aging is also often accompanied by general oral health decline and a reduced ability to swallow, which can affect food choice and intake.
- Many older adults experience mobility constraints, which make it difficult to shop for food, lift heavy jars, open containers, etc.

- As both Wellman and Kinsella mentioned, low income is prevalent in aging populations, making it difficult for many older adults to access high quality foods (i.e., because those foods tend to be more expensive).

A Modified Food Guide Pyramid for Older Adults

Because of the changing dietary needs of older adults, Tucker's colleagues at the Jean Meyer USDA HRNCA developed what they termed the Modified Food Pyramid for older adults (Russell et al., 1999) (Figure 5-1). Key modifications to the original USDA Food Guide Pyramid include placement of water at the bottom of the pyramid because many older adults do not drink enough water to stay hydrated, and placement of a flag at the top of the pyramid indicating the need for calcium, vitamin D, and vitamin B_{12} supplements because many older adults do not get enough of these nutrients in a standard diet. After an update to the Food Guide Pyramid took place for the general population, Tucker's colleagues also created a new Modified MyPyramid for older adults with illustrated examples of healthful foods in each food group (Lichtenstein et al., 2008) (Figure 5-2). Key modifications to the original MyPyramid include the addition of examples of physical

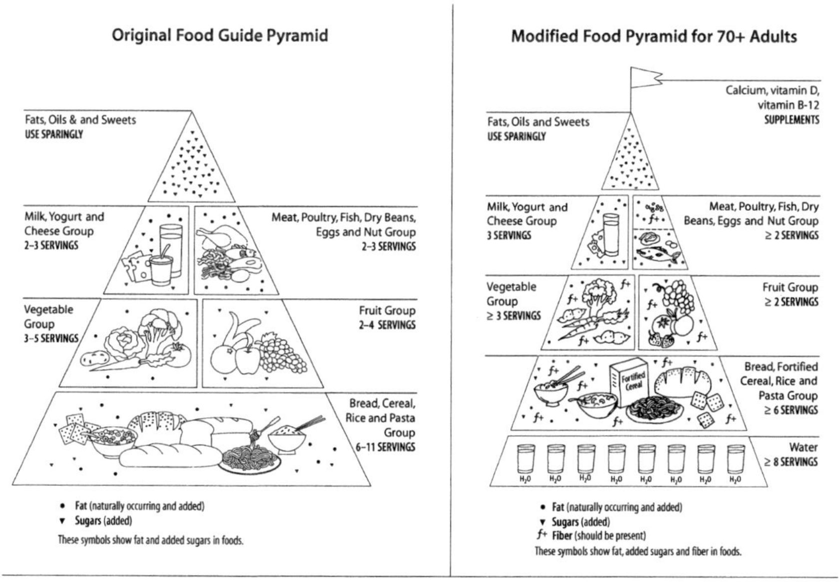

FIGURE 5-1 The original Food Guide Pyramid and the modified Food Guide Pyramid for adults more than 70 years of age.
SOURCE: Russell et al., 1999.

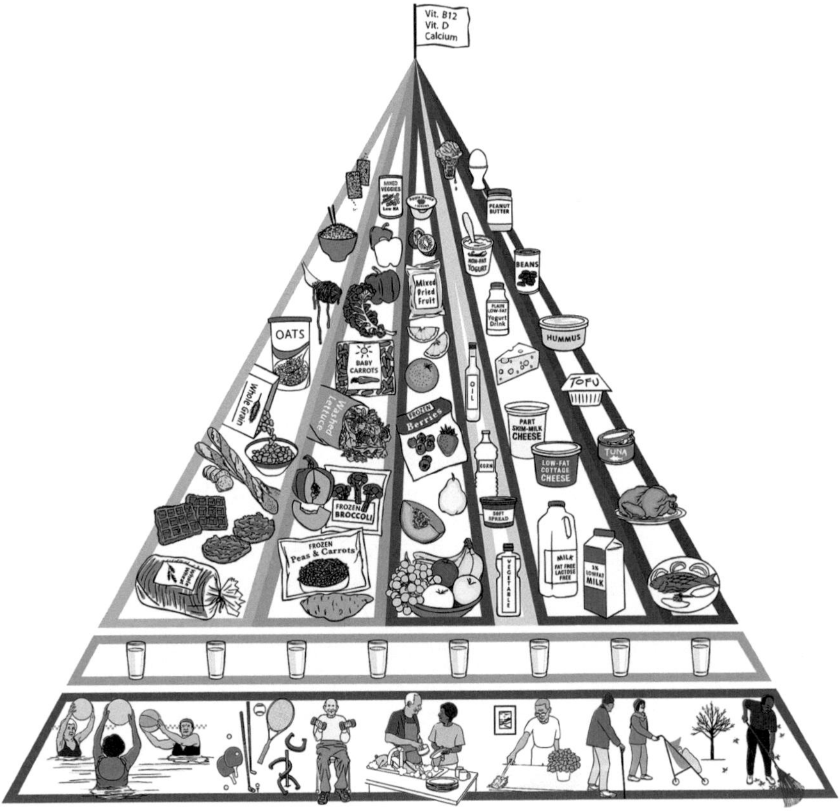

FIGURE 5-2 A modified MyPyramid for adults more than 70 years of age.
SOURCE: Lichtenstein et al., 2008.

activity at the bottom of the pyramid. Greater physical activity allows for intake of larger quantities of food, which in turn increases the likelihood that all of the necessary nutrients will be consumed. Also, physical activity helps maintain muscle mass with aging.

Dietary Patterns of Older Adults

Of course, not all older adults follow the guidelines of the modified MyPyramid. Tucker discussed the variety of ways that older adults eat. She and her colleagues have been examining dietary patterns in older adults as part of the Baltimore Longitudinal Study on Aging.[1] They identified

[1] The Baltimore Longitudinal Study on Aging is a National Institute on Aging (NIA) project. For more information, visit the website http://www.grc.nia.nih.gov/branches/blsa/blsa.htm.

five eating patterns: "white bread" (people that obtain considerably more energy intake from white bread [16 percent, on average] relative to other patterns), "healthy" (higher energy intake from fruit, high fiber cereal, and whole grain bread), "meat" (higher energy intake from meat and potatoes), "alcohol" (higher energy intake from alcohol), and "sweets" (higher energy intake from baked sweets) (Newby et al., 2003). As just one example of how diet affects health, she showed data on waist circumference. Generally, as people age, their weight increases with the rate of increase slowing down over time; most of the gained weight is deposited in the central area of the body. Tucker and her colleagues found that older adults in the "white bread" group experienced a significantly greater increase in weight circumference than older adults in the other eating groups. The "healthy" group showed the least gain in weight circumference.

Protein Intake

Tucker spent much of the remainder of her talk focusing on specific components of the diet, beginning with protein intake. The issue of protein intake in older adults is controversial. She explained that while some experts warn that higher protein intake could be harmful because it could increase the risk of toxicity or impaired renal function, recent research suggests that moderately high protein intake is necessary for maintaining nitrogen balance and offsetting age-related lower energy intake, decreased protein synthetic efficiency, and impaired insulin action. Current recommendations (IOM, 2005) actually call for the same protein intake in both older and younger adults. Even so, according to 2003–2004 data from the National Health and Nutrition Examination Survey (NHANES), about 6 percent of men at the age of 71 and above and about 4 to 6 percent of women above the age of 50 are not meeting the recommended intake levels.

As an example of recent evidence implicating the importance of protein intake, Houston et al. (2008) show that among men and women with sarcopenia[2] and between the ages of 70 and 79, individuals with the highest protein intake lost the least amount of lean muscle mass over a three-year period. Tucker explained that the greater the proportional loss of lean muscle mass, the greater the proportion of fat mass, and the greater the risk of metabolic imbalances and related chronic conditions. Also, loss of lean muscle mass increases the likelihood of falling. She stated that maintaining muscle mass in older adults is one of the most important preventative health steps that can be taken.

In another study, contrary to expectations, Tucker and colleagues found that higher protein intake was associated with lower bone loss (Hannan et

[2] Sarcopenia is the degenerative loss of muscle mass and strength that occurs with aging; muscle mass as a proportion of total body mass decreases.

al., 2000). In the past, based on results from short-term clinical studies, it was generally believed that higher protein intake leads to calcium loss in the urine, which in turn contributes to bone loss.

Other Macronutrients

Tucker briefly described the role of other macronutrients, namely omega-3 fatty acids and fiber, in maintaining health during aging. Dietary fiber is known to be important for maintaining intestinal health and protecting against heart disease and other metabolic conditions. With lipids, the concern with older adults is not too much total fat or too much saturated fat, as it is with younger adults, rather too few omega-3 fatty acids. Epidemiological studies have found that higher intakes of omega-3 fatty acids provide greater protection against many conditions, including cardiovascular events (e.g. arrhythmias, cardiac death, recurrent myocardial infarction), diabetes, and cognitive decline. The problem is that omega-3 fatty acids are very limited in the standard diet, with the main sources being fatty fish, flax seeds, and walnuts. Moreover, the omega-3 fatty acid obtained from flax seeds and walnuts is different than what can be obtained from fatty fish and may not be as beneficial. The health effects associated with this group of fatty acids are an important area of current investigation. Tucker stated that it is unclear whether supplements can provide the same benefits.

Both of these macronutrients are far from adequate in the diets of most older adults. For example, an ongoing study of older Puerto Rican adults in the Boston area has shown that about 40 percent of adults between the ages of 51 and 70 and about 70 percent of adults age 71 and older have omega-3 fatty acid intakes above the Adequate Intake (AI)[3] for n-3 polyunsaturated fatty acids.[4] About 10 percent of 51–70 year-olds and 40 percent of adults 71 and older have dietary intake levels above the AI for fiber. The AIs were established by the Institute of Medicine (IOM, 2005).

---

[3] An Adequate Intake (AI) was developed because of inadequate scientific evidence to determine an Estimated Average Requirement (EAR). The AI is a recommended average daily nutrient intake level based on observed or experimentally determined approximations or estimates of nutrient intake by a group (or groups) of apparently healthy people that are assumed to be adequate. Mean usual intake greater than the AI implies a low prevalence of inadequate intakes, especially when the AI is based on the mean intake of a healthy group.

[4] Omega-3 fatty acids do not specifically have an AI and are instead included in the AI for n-3 polyunsaturated fatty acids. The omega-3 fatty acids DHA and EPA contribute approximately 10 percent of the total n-3 fatty acid intake (IOM, 2005).

Micronutrients

In almost every dietary survey conducted over the past few decades, older adults have inadequate intakes of some essential micronutrients. Moreover, subsets of older adults are often at greater risk of certain micronutrient deficiencies. For example, Non-Hispanic black and low-income older adults typically experience micronutrient intake levels lower than the 1989 Recommended Dietary Allowances (RDA)[5] compared to other groups (Weimer, 1997).

According to 2005–2006 NHANES data, 92 percent of adults over the age of 51 years are below the Estimated Average Requirement (EAR)[6] for vitamin E; 67 percent are below the magnesium EAR; 46 percent are below the vitamin C EAR; 33 percent are below the zinc EAR; and 32 percent are below the vitamin B_6 EAR. Only 14.6 percent are above the AI for calcium (1,200 mg), which Tucker stated is high and controversial. She described in more detail three of these nutrients: vitamin E, vitamin B_6, and magnesium.

Vitamin E. Tucker mentioned Meydani's earlier discussion about vitamin E and the important role that it plays as an antioxidant and in maintaining immune function. She stated that the only straightforward way to meet the currently very high RDA of 15 mg of α-tocopherol is to include nuts and seeds, like almonds or sunflower seeds, in the diet and that there are other important tocopherols in other foods that are being overlooked. Partially because of the difficulties in obtaining sufficient levels of vitamin E through diet, many people are taking vitamin E supplements. Data from the Jackson Heart Study show, however, that concentrations of certain tocopherols are actually lower in people taking supplements (Talegawkar et al., 2007). In particular, γ-tocopherol concentrations in people taking α-tocopherol supplements were half of what they were in people not taking supplements, because the two forms compete with each other. It is not clear what the implications of this exchange are, although some experts believe that loss of γ-tocopherol may somehow contribute to DNA damage. Tucker emphasized that the larger problem is that negative consequences can occur when supplements are used as a substitute for food.

Vitamin B_6. Tucker explained that vitamin B_6 is important for numerous metabolic reactions in the body, with inadequacies sometimes leading to

[5] The Recommended Dietary Allowance (RDA) is an estimate of the daily average dietary intake that meets the nutrient needs of nearly all (97–98 percent) healthy members of a particular life stage and gender group.

[6] The Estimated Average Requirement (EAR) is the average daily nutrient intake level estimated to meet the requirement of half of the healthy individuals in a particular life stage and gender group. It is used to examine the prevalence of nutrient inadequacy in groups.

high homocysteine concentrations and impaired immune function. Vitamin B_6 deficiencies have also been associated with cognitive function decline and depression, both of which are common problems in older adults. Data from the Massachusetts Hispanic Elderly Study show a high prevalence of low vitamin B_6 blood concentrations among both Hispanic and non-Hispanic whites, with 30 percent of Hispanics and 28 percent of non-Hispanic whites having blood concentrations less than 30 nmol/L, and 16 percent of Hispanics and 11 percent of non-Hispanic whites having blood concentrations less than 20 nmol/L (Merete et al., 2008). Data from the Normative Aging Study show that individuals in the lowest tertile of vitamin B_6 concentration have significant loss in cognitive ability over five years, while individuals with the highest vitamin B_6 concentrations showed no loss (Tucker et al., 2005).

Magnesium. Tucker noted only that data from the Framingham Study show that magnesium and potassium are also very important (along with calcium) for maintaining bone health. This means that fruits and vegetables, which people have not associated with bone health in the past (as Tucker said, "it was all about dairy"), are in fact important.

Vitamin B_{12}. The same 2005–2006 NHANES data indicate that very few people age 51 and older (16 percent) are below the EAR for vitamin B_{12}, although there are some subsets of the older population whose intake levels are lower than others (Kwan et al., 2002). Importantly, even though most older adults consume enough vitamin B_{12}, it nonetheless remains a serious problem in the aging population because it is so poorly absorbed due to decreased stomach acidity. Many widely prescribed and over-the-counter acid blocking drugs also block the ability to absorb vitamin B_{12}. Data from the Framingham Offspring Study (Tucker et al., 2000) showed that 8 percent of vitamin B_{12} supplement users still had low concentrations of B_{12} in their blood (0.250 μmol/L), and 20 percent of non-supplement users had low concentrations. Low vitamin B_{12} concentrations in older adults create a serious problem, as deficiencies can lead to a variety of serious nerve-related effects, including peripheral neuropathy, balance disturbances, cognitive disturbances, and ultimately physical disability (e.g., see Healton et al., 1991). Inadequate concentrations of vitamin B_{12} also lead to high homocysteine concentrations and a greater risk of heart disease. New findings also show an association between lower vitamin B_{12} concentrations and greater loss of bone density (Tucker et al., 2005).

Other studies suggest additional vulnerabilities to compromised nutrient status among older adults (e.g., Lichtenstein et al., 2008). Lichtenstein and colleagues (2008) also showed that folate and sodium, on the other hand, are overconsumed by older adults. While overconsumption of sodium among older adults has been well known for a long time Tucker remarked folate overconsumption is an interesting story.

Folate. Folic acid was added to the food supply as a way to protect against neural tube defects, with the goal of reaching women at childbearing age before they get pregnant. However, researchers have since identified several possible adverse effects of high folic acid in the food supply, including accelerated effects of vitamin B_{12} deficiency (while folate masks B_{12} deficiency by covering up the anemia, it also drives pathways that make the B_{12} deficiency worse), an increased risk of some cancers (while folic acid from food can be protective against cancer, large amounts of folic acid from supplements or fortified foods can accumulate in the blood), and an increased risk of cognitive decline (again, folic acid from food can protect against cognitive decline because of its important role in DNA methylation, but large amounts of folic acid may be detrimental).

Vitamin D. Tucker explained that older adults are at high risk of vitamin D inadequacy because of limited sources of vitamin D in the diet (fortified milk, fatty fishes), less exposure to sunlight, a decreased capacity to synthesize vitamin D in the skin even when exposure to sunlight is plentiful, and a decreased capacity of the kidneys to convert vitamin D into its active form. In the past, the focus with vitamin D was on calcium absorption and metabolism and bone health. Now, vitamin D has been proposed to be associated with many neurological and other chronic conditions. Tucker shared data from an ongoing study of an older Puerto Rican population near Boston showing that only 18 percent of adults between 51 and 70 years old have intakes above the AI and just 8 percent of adults age 71 and older have intakes above the AI. In a study of homebound elders, Buell et al. (2009) found that more than 60 percent of their study population had insufficient vitamin D concentrations in their blood (less than 20 ng/mL), and more than 50 percent had less than 400 international units (IU) intake per day. When the data were examined by race, the researchers found that about 69 percent of non-black elders had vitamin D deficiency (defined in this study as less than 10 ng/mL), compared to about 80 percent of black elders. Buell and colleagues (2009) also identified associations between vitamin D deficiency and several different measures of cognitive function with the interesting exception of memory.

Dietary Variety

In conclusion, Tucker said that "one of the most important things we can do for the aging population" is ensure good dietary intake. Important risk nutrients include protein; omega-3 fatty acids; dietary fiber; vitamins B_6, B_{12}, and E; calcium; magnesium; and potassium. Many older adults are not getting enough of these nutrients. On the other hand, too many older adults are getting too much folate and sodium. She remarked the best way to ensure good dietary intake is by increasing intake of whole grains, fruits and vegetables, fish, nuts, lean protein sources, and low-fat dairy and decreasing intake of refined grains and highly processed foods. Tucker emphasized the importance of complexity in the diet and referred to a study suggesting higher dietary variety is associated with overall better nutritional status and better health outcomes in frail elderly people (Bernstein et al., 2002). The challenge is getting good quality foods to this population.

FUNCTIONAL FOODS AND AGING POPULATIONS

Presenter: Stephen Barnes

Barnes began by remarking that he would be talking about functional foods and some of the challenges around bioavailability of active compounds in functional foods.

What Is a Functional Food?

Barnes explained that functional foods were not specifically defined in the Federal Food, Drug, and Cosmetic (FDC) Act of 1938. Instead, he referred to a 1994 IOM definition of functional food: a "food or food ingredient that may provide a health benefit beyond the traditional nutrients it contains" (IOM, 1994). Many functional foods are conventional foods, that is, foods that were foods even before the concept of a functional food was generated; often they contain specific GRAS (Generally Recognized as Safe) components with known benefits. However, anytime a health-promoting claim is made about an item that is not related to the item's "nutritive" value, the item is considered a supplement and thereby falls under the provisions of the Dietary Supplement Health and Education Act (DSHEA). If a claim is made that relates to disease treatment or prevention, the item is considered a drug.

Barnes's interest in functional foods stemmed from his interest in soy and the fact that the chemistry of isoflavones varies among different types of soy foods. In Asia, soy is consumed largely in the form of miso, which is a fermented form of soybean; and soymilk and tofu, which are extracted from heated soybean. In the United States, on the other hand, soy is consumed largely in the form of textured vegetable protein, which is processed differently than the common Asian soy foods and therefore has a different composition (i.e., it is processed through dry heat, not fermentation or hot water extraction). In fermented and hot water extracted products, the soy isoflavones are not only converted into readily absorbable forms of genistein (i.e., 6-hydroxy and 8-hydroxy genistein), they also contain added chemical groups that make them more bioactive. With dry heat, on the other hand, the isoflavones are converted into an acetyl glucoside form of genistein that is not absorbed very well until it reaches the lower gut. Barnes questioned whether the benefits of fermented or hot water extracted soy functional foods exist with these other dry heat products.

In addition to isoflavonoids in soy (and also kudzu), some of the other most common bioactive components of functional foods include fiber (in whole grains), carotenoids (in carrots, tomatoes and green vegetables), allicin (in garlic), flavonoids (in fruits and green tea), sulforaphane (in broccoli sprouts), and omega-3 fatty acids (in wild fish).

Functional Foods for Aging Populations

Barnes stated that these and other bioactive compounds could be used to create functional foods for older adults that improve or maintain taste and smell, digestion, brain health, the immune system, bone and joint health, cardiovascular health, gut flora (i.e., probiotic foods), and eye health. A recent survey indicates that many older adults are in fact eating more fruits and vegetables as they age because of these and other potential health-promoting (i.e., functional) benefits (Shatenstein et al., 2003). As for dietary supplements, the top 20 sellers in 2008 are listed in Table 5-1.

Barnes emphasized the importance of considering whether foods are in a form that older adults can actually digest. Not only do many older adults not have adequate teeth, they could be experiencing problems related to impaired acid production (e.g., due to medications that interfere with acid production), or other physiological changes such as those discussed in Chapter 3.

TABLE 5-1 Top-Selling Dietary Supplements in 2008

Dietary Supplement	
Cranberry	Green tea
Soy	Evening primrose
Garlic	Valerian
Saw palmetto	Horny goat weed
Gingko	Grape seed
Echinacea	Elderberry
Milk thistle	Bilberry
St. John's Wort	Ginger
Ginseng	Horse chestnut seed
Black cohosh	Yohimbe

SOURCE: Cavaliere et al., 2009.

Bioavailability: Absorption, Distribution, Metabolism, and Excretion (ADME) in Older Adults

Barnes recalled how once, as a student, he had entered a pub late in the evening and observed a group of "little old ladies" knitting and drinking stout. He realized later that the women were probably not drinking the stout to drink stout, but rather because stout is very nutritious for older adults. A pint of stout has only 200 calories, is low in sodium, and is rich in vitamin B_6, iron, and flavonoids. He described stout as a "very good soup." Moreover, it is easy to digest. Stout is a great example of how physical form matters. He stated that foods are generally much better than dietary supplements in terms of bioavailability, because the bioactives are generally much more dispersed among the food particles and therefore more likely to be absorbed by the body. Bioavailability of purified compounds (i.e., a dietary supplement) is very dependent on the physical properties of those compounds, and many dietary supplements are simply not very well absorbed.

He used flavonoids in foods to illustrate how bioavailability is impacted by the physiology of the gastrointestinal (GI) tract, beginning in the oral cavity where pre-hydrolysis (i.e., pre-digestion) dissolves some fats and sends signals to the rest of the GI system that "food is coming." Then, in the stomach, there may be some hydrolysis, although Barnes is unsure to what extent. Small intestine metabolism, however, is definitely very important, with lactase and other intestinal enzymes preparing (hydrolyzing) the flavonoid glycosides[7] for enterohepatic circulation (i.e., the compound passes through either the small intestine or large intestine wall, enters the liver where other metabolic processes occur, and then reenters the small intestine). Flavonoids not absorbed in the small intestine are metabolized by microflora in the colon, where they undergo considerable structural modifications. In the colon, bioavailability is impacted by transit time and bacterial composition, with a faster transit time leading to less enterohepatic circulation (and therefore less metabolism and absorption) and the presence of certain bacterial populations also affecting metabolism. Changes in any of these organs, as well as changes in kidney or renal function, can impact bioavailability. Importantly, drug interactions could occur at any point along this pathway, also impacting bioavailability.

[7] All flavonoids, except flavanols, are found in glycosylated forms in foods. This is a key factor influencing bioavailability because in these native forms, most flavonoids cannot be absorbed (D'Archivio et al., 2010).

Conclusion

In conclusion, Barnes echoed what other speakers had emphasized: Optimizing nutrition is important. In fact, that is the rationale for functional foods. However, depending on what type of processing methods are used to make the functional food, some of the potential health benefits may not be as great as they are in other, differently processed foods because of reduced bioavailability. In other words, not all soy products are necessarily alike with respect to their health-promoting benefits, because of how different processing technologies alter bioavailability of the compounds that confer those benefits. Moreover, the fact that aging alters the properties of all of various organs that handle bioactive compounds in food creates another major challenge to formulating and providing health-promoting functional foods to older adults. With respect to drug-food interactions, which could occur at any point along the GI pathway and impact bioavailability, Barnes said that is "something we don't know enough about."

NUTRITIONAL MODULATION OF AGING AND AGE-ASSOCIATED DISEASES BY CALORIC RESTRICTION

Presenter: Luigi Fontana

Fontana began by defining aging as "the progressive accumulation of cell/tissue/organ damage with time." He emphasized that aging is a lifetime process and not something "kicking in when you are 65," which means that how people behave (e.g., eat) when they are young and middle-aged matters. The accumulation of damage is due to failure of maintenance and repair mechanisms to completely protect against damage, leading to progressive decline in function and structure and eventually death. Importantly, chronic diseases accelerate the accumulation of damage.

Is Aging Preventable?

While aging is not preventable, there are interventions that can slow it. The best characterized of these is caloric restriction (CR) without malnutrition. Fontana said hundreds of studies in yeast, worms, and mice and rats have shown that CR can slow aging, with about 10 percent CR increasing maximal life span by as much as 50 percent. As an example, Fontana showed data from Weindruch and Walford (1982) and Weindruch and Sohal (1997) indicating the impact of CR on the lifespan of rodents (Figure 5-3).

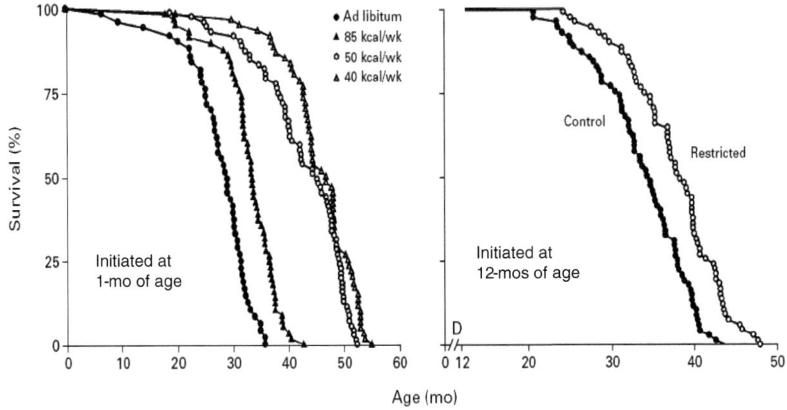

FIGURE 5-3 Survival of rodents placed on ad libitum versus calorie restricted diets. This evidence suggests that long term caloric restriction without malnutrition may extend healthspan and maximal lifespan in rodents.
SOURCES: Weindruch and Walford, 1982; Weindruch and Sohal, 1997.

Murine models of longevity include

- Ames and Snell dwarf mice,
- growth hormone receptor knock-out (KO) mice,
- insulin-like growth factor-1 (IGF-1) receptor deficient mice,
- klotho overexpressing mice,
- fat insulin receptor KO mice,
- insulin receptor substrate 1 KO mice,
- brain insulin receptor substrate 2 KO mice,
- ribosomal S6 protein kinase 1 KO mice,
- p66shc KO mice,
- type 5 adenylyl cyclase KO mice, and
- Ang II type 1 KO mice.

Are Chronic Diseases Associated with Aging Preventable?

Despite the current "epidemic of obesity" in the United States and associations between excessive adiposity and cardiovascular disease mortality (Calle et al., 1999), cancer mortality (Hu et al., 2004) and other conditions (Willet et al., 1999), Fontana said that his interest in CR is not weight loss. Rather, he is interested in what a 20 or 30 year old man or woman who wants to live a longer and, more importantly, healthier life, can do. He defined healthy aging as the ability of human beings to remain physically and mentally healthy, happy and creative, empowered, active, contributing, and independent for as long as possible. His questions are (1) What interventions, even among lean individuals, promote healthy aging?, and (2)Are chronic diseases associated with aging preventable?

Data from CR in animals suggest that not only do calorie restricted animals live longer lives, they also are more likely to die without any pathologies. In one study, none of the CR animals showed any signs of pathological lesions upon autopsy, whereas only six percent of the animals on a typical diet (i.e., non-CR diet) showed no signs of pathology (Shimokawa et al. 1993). Subsequently, Colman et al. (2009) suggested that CR "works" not only in mice and rats but also in primates. Rhesus monkeys fed a 30 percent CR diet starting in middle age demonstrated a 50 percent reduction in cardiovascular disease mortality and a 50 percent reduction in cancer mortality. Fontana said that the implications of this study are "huge," because both the CR and control animals were fed a very healthful diet. As far as extension in maximal life span goes, the researchers will not know for another 10 years if CR animals live longer.

He mentioned another study demonstrating even among lean animals with the same body weight, only those fed a CR diet had an extended maximal life span (Holloszy, 1997). Exercise did not increase maximal life span; it only increased average life span, presumably by preventing excessive adiposity and the type of metabolic alterations that typically accompany excessive adiposity (e.g., type 2 diabetes). Only CR slowed down "intrinsic aging."

Then he discussed a study that he has been involved with for the past two years, where he and his colleagues are examining the effects of CR without malnutrition in a group of healthy volunteers between the ages of 35 and 82. The CR participants (n = 32) are eating 100 percent of their Reference Daily Intake (RDI) for each nutrient and approximately 1800 calories daily. They have been doing this for eight years, on average. The first control group (n = 32) is a group of age and sex-matched U.S. athletes that are equally lean because they are running about 50 miles a week and eating about 2,000 calories daily. The second control group (n = 32) is a group of matched sedentary individuals eating a typical American diet. The researchers are examining the effects of these three different diets (i.e., CR participants, exercisers, and sedentary participants) on body mass index, body fat, hormone levels, glucose tolerance and insulin action, cardiometabolic risk factors, carotid artery thickness, and arterial elasticity. Only published data are presented here. Fontana et al. (2004) found that CR practitioners had significantly lower serum concentrations of several risk factors, including lower total and low-density lipoprotein (LDL) cholesterol, fasting glucose, C-reactive protein, and blood pressure.

Fontana et al. (2009) found that both CR and exercisers had significantly lower fasting glucose and insulin levels than the sedentary group.

Insulin is a risk factor for cardiovascular disease and cancer, and it has been implicated in aging. However, when challenged with a glucose load, the athletes did much better than the CR individuals, suggesting that exercise is much more powerful than CR in preventing type 2 diabetes.

Fontana remarked that clearly hormones and growth factors play a major role in modulating aging in humans. The same changes that have been observed in humans (i.e., reduction in inflammation, insulin, and total testosterone) also occur in mice, rats, and primates, with one important difference. In rats, long-term CR reduces serum IGF-1 concentration by 40 percent (Breece et al., 1991). In humans, however, long-term CR does not reduce serum IGF-1 concentrations (Fontana et al., 2008). IGF-1 is a risk factor for premenopausal breast cancer, prostate cancer, and colon cancer, so the higher the IGF-1 concentration, the greater the risk of developing these cancers (Chan et al., 1998; Hankinson et al., 1998). Not only is IGF-1 a major player in cancer, Fontana said that it is also probably important in the aging process itself.

The Importance of Protein

While CR may not reduce serum IGF-1 concentration in humans, moderate protein restriction does. Fontana and his colleagues realized this when they observed that a group of strict vegans in the study described in Fontana et al. (2008) had significantly lower IGF-1 than either controls or people on a CR diet. The average American obtains about 15 to 16 percent of calories from protein. People on the CR diet had a very high protein diet, obtaining about 24 percent of calories from protein. The vegans obtained only about 10 percent of calories from protein. During the course of the study, Fontana asked some of the CR individuals to go on reduced protein diet, after which their IGF-1 serum levels dropped 25 percent, suggesting that protein restriction is more important than calories in reducing IGF-1.

Noting that the Recommended Dietary Allowance (RDA) for protein is 0.83 g/kg per day and that many people are consuming much more than this (Rand et al., 2003), Fontana challenged workshop participants to consider that while nitrogen balance data may be suggesting that older adults need more protein, not less, IGF-1 data suggest otherwise. Fontana and colleagues are currently studying protein restriction (not just CR) in both animals and humans.

Conclusion

In conclusion, Fontana stated that other factors besides CR, and possibly protein restriction, also affect aging. For example, exercise is very important. Likewise, phytochemical intake may impact antiaging pathways independent of CR and other interventions. Moreover, CR is not necessarily always beneficial. Too much restriction can have detrimental effects and may even lead to death. Plus, various factors such as age, sex, and genetic predisposition might also make a difference. For example, Fontana said that starting a CR diet at the age of 65 is probably not a good idea. CR should be started at an earlier age to control body weight and avoid increased abdominal fat, though Fontana did not specify an age range.

FORMULATING FOR AGING BOOMER CONSUMERS

Presenter: Jim Kirkwood

Kirkwood began by describing his role at General Mills as somebody who connects the science with something that people actually want to eat. He asks the question: Since consumers don't understand much of the science around nutrition and food safety (i.e., the science that is being discussed during this workshop), what drives their decision-making? He remarked that most of his talk would revolve around efforts that General Mills food developers and creators are making to understand what drives aging boomer consumers' food choices.

General Mills is the world's sixth largest food company, with products marketed in more than 100 countries. Aging consumers are very important to General Mills because of the fast rate of growth in the aging population. Kirkwood said that 65 percent of the estimated future growth for General Mills will come from aging boomer consumers.[8]

Kirkwood posed the question, "Who are these aging boomer consumers?" He asked the audience to raise their hands if they thought that old age "starts" at 45. Several people raised their hands. When asked if old age starts at 55, a few more people raised their hands. When asked if it starts at 65, many more people raised their hands. At 75, everybody had their hands raised. He said that if General Mills were to build food products for aging consumers, nobody would buy them, because nobody is aging in his or her own mind. In a survey of 2,969 adults conducted by the Pew Research Center, 65 percent of respondents 75 and older did not consider themselves "old." When asked at what age one becomes old, on average, 18–29 year-olds said 60, 30–49 year-olds said 69, and 50–64 year-olds said 72.

Kirkwood then posed the question, "What do aging consumers care about?" He emphasized that while scientific evidence is very important from a food development perspective, consumers are driven by other fac-

[8] Kirkwood cited Nielson Scantrack and HomeScan, BCS Analysis, as the source of these facts.

tors. He and his team have identified five key areas of concern among aging boomer consumers: (1) physical vitality; (2) mental acuity; (3) legacy (i.e., what people are going to leave for their families and in the world, how they will be remembered); (4) financial security; and (5) community (e.g., many people fear being alone as they get older). Of these, mental acuity is the biggest consumer worry. People assume that medicines would be available for physical health problems and that family and other sources would be available for financial assistance, if necessary, but it would be very difficult to deal with loss of mental acuity.

Kirkwood asked, "What do these questions have to do with food?" He explained, "Food is only an enabler for the things that really matter to consumers. . . . If we can tie food to what matters, then we will be able to inject good things into their lives." If food developers do not relate their products to what is important for consumers, then consumers will not use those products. For boomers in particular, compromise is not an option. He said, "Boomers do not want to give up anything. They want it all."

In order to relate products to those factors that are important to consumers, companies must do two things according to Kirkwood: (1) comprehensively understand aging consumers' needs, and (2) translate that understanding into food solutions that consumers want, need, and can afford.

Kirkwood then showed a short film, *Project Goldie*, describing the results of ethnography studies that General Mills has conducted as a way to understand baby boomer consumer values. The video demonstrated that while food is important, there are many other factors besides food that are also important to people's lives. In particular, there are six key needs of aging consumers: (1) health and wellness, (2) care for others, (3) grandchildren, (4) connections, (5) life experiences, and (6) small households.

Product Development

Product development—that is, translating aging consumers' needs into products on the shelf—is a very complex, time-consuming process. It involves everything from "culinary creation" (i.e., making a food that tastes good) to ensuring microbiological stability and regulatory compliance. Kirkwood said that everything that goes into product development can be broken down into four essential "elements":

- *Form* (i.e., channel, product form, and package configuration). Form is a key element of the decision-making that goes on around how a product is going to be formulated. For example, will the product be refrigerated, frozen, or shelf stable? Is it something that consumers will want to carry with them? Is it something that people will enjoy preparing for their grandchildren? With respect to package configuration, will the product be single-serve? For aging boomer consumers, ease of use and legibility of preparation instructions are additional considerations (e.g., Kirkwood referred to Brody's description of the packaging industry's efforts to develop new types of easy-to-open packages).

- *Function* (i.e., safety, benefit delivery, and nutritional delivery). Function is another key consideration, with the primary goal being to ensure that a product is safe regardless of consumer need. With respect to benefit delivery, if a product is designed to deliver a specific benefit, that benefit must be validated by science and the necessary ingredient(s) put into the product in a way that ensures bioavailability and that the product is delivering what the package/company claims that it is delivering. For older adults, this means that the health benefit is validated with the targeted age group and that the products actually deliver those benefits specifically to older adults. Nutritional delivery refers to the fact that benefits aside, foods deliver nutrients; therefore, the product in question should be delivering the nutrients it is supposed to be delivering, particularly those nutrients with intake levels that are of greatest concern among older adults.
- *Appeal* (i.e., taste, texture, and appearance). If a product does not taste or look good, people will not eat it, regardless of its contents. Product development involves extensive sensory work to ensure that the intended benefits are delivered. For aging boomer consumers, additional considerations include vibrancy, potency, and consistency. Vibrancy is the way a food is experienced, for example, its appearance or mouthfeel. Potency refers to a taste profile that hits the "sweet spot" for older adults, especially given that the sense of taste changes with aging. Consistency refers to the texture of a food and the need to develop foods that are not, for example, too crunchy or too hard.
- *Affordability* (i.e., raw materials, manufacturability, distribution). This is a huge concern, especially in today's economic climate and especially for aging boomer consumers. Product developers must determine an acceptable price point for the target audience and then design development so that the product can meet that price point. They do this by optimizing raw material usage, working with suppliers to ensure a cost-effective supply chain, and minimizing manufacturing and distribution costs. Also, unit size is important. As people age, they tend to cook only for themselves (i.e., two-people households).

The Fiber One Bar: An Example of a Product That Works

Kirkwood used the Fiber One bar as an example of a product developed for aging boomer consumers. The Fiber One bar is designed to meet the Health and Wellness need category (i.e., one of the six need categories identified in the film *Project Goldie*). Nine out of ten Americans do not get the recommended amount of whole grains and fiber, and consumers know this. They know they need to eat more fiber in order to feel better, but they also want to get that fiber in a way that suits their lifestyles. It can't be something that does not taste good, and it has to be something that they know is "working." Kirkwood described how he and his team at General Mills considered all four key elements of product development (form, function, appeal, and affordability) as they made decisions regarding the concept and development plan for the Fiber One bar:

- *Form:* They developed a product that was shelf stable, in easy-to-eat bar form, and in a single serve pouch, because they knew that people wanted to be able to carry the product with them.
- *Function:* They developed a product that delivered 35 percent of the daily fiber recommendation to the target population (i.e., older boomer consumers), had a healthful nutrient profile (e.g., low salt, low fat), and had simple ingredients (i.e., ingredients that consumers recognize, like nuts and wheat).
- *Appeal:* They developed a product with "unexpected great taste," a soft chewy texture, and a natural appearance.
- *Affordability:* They developed a product with a novel fiber that lowered the cost of the bar from $10 to an affordable price, and formulated it to fit existing factory systems to minimize manufacturing costs.

In conclusion, Kirkwood remarked that the end result is a product that, since launch, has provided nearly 10 billion grams of fiber to the American diet. The Fiber One bar is an example of a product that has "clearly intervened in Americans' lives."

PANEL DISCUSSION ON IMPLICATIONS FOR REGULATORS, EDUCATORS, AND THE FOOD INDUSTRY

The four presentations prompted questions about recommended maximum daily nutrient intakes, the importance of protein in older adults' diets, hypothesized mechanisms that might explain the effect of caloric restriction (CR) on aging, and drug-nutrient interactions.

Recommended Maximum Daily Intakes

An audience member asked whether there was any sort of "fudge factor" in Dietary Reference Intakes (DRI) to compensate for variation in sensitivity. The questioner expressed concern about communicating some of the statistics about nutrient intake. For example, if 92 percent of the population has a less than adequate intake of a particular nutrient, how can that information be communicated in such a way that people will not automatically think that they are probably among that 92 percent and therefore are probably going to suffer the consequences? Tucker explained that the RDA is designed to meet the estimated requirement for almost all healthy individuals, which means that many people do not need to meet the RDA. DRI values also contain an Estimated Average Requirement (EAR) which can be used to assess prevalence of inadequacy. She suggested that when 70 percent or more of a group has values below the EAR that there may be reason for concern.

The Importance of Protein in Older Adults' Diets

Another audience member asked Tucker if she was aware of any studies on associations between amino acids, specifically branched-chain amino acids, and sarcopenia. Tucker replied that most of her work was with whole foods and that she was unaware of any studies on specific amino acids. Barnes remarked that he had recently attended a session on food peptides at a World Food Congress and that, while largely ignored in the United States, many Asian scientists are studying bioactivity of specific amino acids and peptides in foods.

The Mechanism of the Effect of Caloric Restriction on Longevity

Fontana was asked about his thoughts on the mechanism of CR's effect on improved health and life expectancy. Fontana replied that there is a great deal of research focused on identifying and understanding which mechanisms are mediating the antiaging effects of CR without malnutrition. While data from genetic animal model studies on longevity are filling some gaps in knowledge, he stated that the major mechanisms are unknown. So far, six different animal models for longevity suggest that the IGF-1 pathway is important. Animals with low IGF-1 live longer, healthier lives than animals with high IGF-1, causing Fontana to call IGF-1 "the new frontier." But other animal models of longevity indicate that there are other factors at play, such as catecholamine signaling and angiotensin activity.

Drug-Nutrient Interactions

Finally, Barnes was asked to elaborate on a parenthetical comment he had made before he began his presentation about disagreeing with Greenblatt's view on drug-nutrient interactions. Barnes said that he believes there is much more to drug activity than metabolism and the interaction between a drug and a single metabolizing enzyme. By examining only the way that a drug interacts with "your favorite enzyme" and not, for example, how that drug is transported through the body, results in a "rather narrow viewpoint." Moreover, he emphasized the importance of examining drug-nutrient interactions under the type of stressful physiological conditions that many older adults typically experience.

6

Communicating with Aging Populations

Food Forum member Edward Groth of Groth Consulting Services, Pelham, New York, opened this session by identifying two major challenges to communicating about food safety and nutrition with aging populations. First, having come from a background filled with "miscommunication about toxic chemicals and food safety," he said that communication often fails because while the expert community assumes that all it has to do is "explain the wonderful science . . . and the public will fall in line," this is not the case. Changing behavior is difficult, and it is important to know where the public is coming from. Kirkwood touched on this theme in his presentation during an earlier session, which is summarized in Chapter 5, as did several of the speakers in this session. Second, Groth cautioned that the number of newspapers regularly reporting science has decreased by more than two-thirds over the past 20 years or so, and magazines are "folding left and right." He said that some people have described the current science communication environment as a "science communication crisis."

He then introduced the first of four speakers for this session, Steven Bodhaine of The Futures Company, Chapel Hill, North Carolina. Bodhaine spoke about communication from a consumer perspective, emphasizing the importance of engaging consumers in a personal way. He described the results of a study aimed at understanding what motivates behavior change in older adult consumers. Caroline Smith DeWaal of the Center for Science in the Public Interest (CSPI), Washington, DC, discussed how consumers hear about and respond to food recall messages and outlined lessons learned from recent food recalls. She emphasized the need to consider on-the-spot messaging as a way to reach older adults when urgent food safety information needs to be communicated. William Hallman of the Food Policy Institute (FPI) at Rutgers University, New Brunswick, New Jersey, discussed results of several FPI surveys aimed at understanding how people interpret and respond to food recalls. He echoed other calls to make food safety communication personal, and he also emphasized the importance of sending specific messages about what actions consumers should take. Finally, Ronni Chernoff of the Geriatric Research Education and Clinical Center, John L. McClellan Memorial Veterans Hospital, Little Rock, Arkansas, discussed health literacy in general and described key elements of effective written and oral health communication. She emphasized the importance of reinforcing key messages when communicating about food safety and nutrition.

The session ended with a lengthy discussion with the audience. There were many questions about food recall compliance and how to improve food recall communication, the concept of opt-out strategizing (which Bodhaine had mentioned during his talk as a strategy for motivating behavioral change), the concept of "persuade by reason, motivate by emotion" (which Bodhaine had also introduced), the use of symbols to communicate food safety information, and the challenge of sending simple messages about complicated situations.

CONSUMER DESIRES, NEEDS, AND MOTIVATIONS

Presenter: Steven Bodhaine

Bodhaine began by remarking that he hoped his talk would be somewhat provocative and that the ideas and material he would be presenting were based on considerable consumer research: The Futures Company has been tracking consumer behavior for 40 years. He emphasized that health is not the center of most people's lives, and health communication is "competing for attention in a very cluttered world." In fact, he said, "I would submit that we are beyond clutter. We have actually entered an era of market resistance, where consumers are taking active measures to avoid our communication." He argued further, "The era of mass marketing is over. It is dead. We can no longer expect to send a single message and hope that it will have resonance with our target audience."

The 2009 Health and Wellness Segmentation Study

Bodhaine walked the workshop audience through some of what he and his colleagues have learned from their 2009 Health and Wellness Segmentation Study aimed at understanding what motivates behavior change in consumers, particularly around health and wellness. The study was Wave 3 of the Yankelovich Health and Wellness Segmentation Study and included 6,000 U.S. respondents aged 18 and older. Participants were asked to fill out a 50-minute web-based questionnaire, and data were weighted by age, gender, income, education, and ethnicity. The study was based on the notion that people are taking different journeys through life, and understanding those journeys can aid in communicating more effectively and in a way that motivates behavior change.

The study identified six types of journeys:

- *Leading the Way* (traditional, responsible, and proactive): 10 percent of study participants were identified as *Leading the Way*. Health is a core value for these people, and most of them have normal body mass index (BMI), do not smoke, care about what they eat and drink, exercise regularly, and see a physician. Bodhaine described *Leading the Way* people as having an internal locus of control and a future orientation, firmly believing that they can take charge and make a difference both now and in the future. Health communications to *Leading the Way* people work: they listen to messages such as "Be careful with what you eat in order to avoid future incidence of cancer."
- *In It for Fun* (sporty, wealth-oriented, driven): 17 percent of study participants were identified as *In it for Fun*. While *In It for Fun* people exercise, care about their weight, and watch what they eat, though their efforts have nothing to do with health. They value "looking good and feeling fine." Exercise is part of their social fabric. They enjoy competition, and they want to be at the top of their game in order to reach their goals and meet their ambitions. *In It for Fun* people are not motivated by the same messages that *Leading the Way* people are, even though both types espouse healthful lifestyles.
- *Value Independence* (ambitious, hardworking, leisure-less): 19 percent of study participants were identified as *Value Independence*. These are the "do-it-yourselfers," people who have lost faith in science, organized medicine, and the voice of the expert. They are tired of confusing, conflicting, and contradictory messaging, and because they are savvy, they have concluded that they can "do it themselves." They have access to information on the Internet, which they search diligently and judiciously. The challenge is that they are blinded by what they do not know. They have an attitude of profound cynicism. Many *Value Independence* people have a difficult time managing weight. They struggle to find "the solution" that ultimately works.

On average, they each have four chronic conditions. Because they have embraced the value of virtual health and place more confidence in the empathetic voice of a third party than they do in their physician, Bodhaine said that communicating with them poses a "very interesting challenge."

- *I Need a Plan* (traditional, home-oriented, and self-assured): 20 percent of study participants were identified as *I Need a Plan*. Individuals in this "undisciplined" group of people are exceedingly pleasant, Bodhaine said, "absolutely committed to dieting until chocolate cake is served." Whereas *Leading the Way* and *Value Independence* people possess extraordinary internal loci of control, *I Need a Plan* people do not. They go on and off diets and, while willing, "cannot get there alone." They embrace and applaud every bit of nutritional information but do not apply it. Reaching this group of people requires checklists, coaching, follow up, and accountability. People in this group have five chronic conditions each, on average, and obesity is one of their biggest health challenges.
- *Not Right Now* (entertainment, downtime, family): 24 percent of study participants were identified as *Not Right Now*. People in this group tend to be younger and have somebody in their family who, for example, "is 93 years old and has been smoking since she was seven" and with whom they share the same genes. They are generally healthy. Their indifference makes them difficult to reach, and furthermore, they are also ultra-pressed for time, racing about to maintain a professional agenda while also raising young children. They don't feel any sense of urgency to change their behavior, and they view exercise and better nutrition as something that they will pursue when their kids are grown. They respond "more to the stick than to the carrot." They will not change their behavior unless they are absolutely pushed through the door and forced to change.
- *Get Through the Day* (cautious, handy, and cash-strapped): 11 percent of study participants were identified as *Get through the Day*. Most people in this group have struggled with poor health for much of their lives. They average six chronic conditions each. They are very dependent on physicians and other health care professionals. They have tried and stopped many things in an effort to improve their health. Medically, they are an expensive group because of extensive physician interaction and pharmaceutical intervention. Although they want to be in control, they cannot succeed on their own.

Bodhaine reiterated that people are taking different journeys through life and that, when it comes to communication, "one size does not fit all." Importantly, the goal of communication is not just to deliver information. Bodhaine said, "The last thing the consumer needs is more information." Consumers already know that they need to eat better, lose weight, stop smoking, etc., in order to improve their health. In 2005, when the Healthy and Wellness Segmentation Study was first conducted, two-thirds of Americans were identified as overweight, and one-third as obese; statistics that persisted in 2009. This was true despite the fact that the messages to eat better, lose weight, stop smoking, etc. were communicated repeatedly in the intervening years. Why? Bodhaine said, "I would contend that one of the reasons that health is so hard is because life has become so easy. We have to learn how to apply certain tools to get people to move."

Persuade Through Reason, Motivate Through Emotion

While the language of science is persuasive, rarely does the public act in response to scientific information. Bodhaine said, "We persuade by reason, but we motivate through emotion." He used units of measurement on food labels as an example of the type of scientific information that is often meaningless to consumers. While including "serving size" information on labels is a step forward, most consumers do not have any visual cues to understand what the designated serving size actually is. The opt-out 100-calorie packs have also been helpful, as the word "calorie" on a food label means nothing to most consumers. Even if someone eats three or four 100-calorie packs of Oreos, that is better than eating a whole box. Similarly, "grams" means very little to many consumers, with many people not knowing whether a gram is greater or less than an ounce. As a final example, words like "riboflavin" have about as much meaning as words like "octane." Most people know that 93 octane costs more than 87 octane, but beyond that, most consumers have no idea what octane is. Many consumers interpret nutrition information in the same way. They use it to compare (e.g., "This has more than that."), without any real understanding of whether the nutrient or product in question is healthful.

Often, communicating solely on a rational platform is viewed as argumentative and rarely motivates behavior change. Even though there is power in the language of science, communicators often find they need to back away from the science if they want to reach consumers. Bodhaine emphasized that science communicators must link science to emotion. On the other hand, communicating solely on an emotive platform is viewed as communicating "fluff" and being manipulative. The challenge is to connect the science with something that is personally relevant to the consumer and then deliver the information in a way that is going to motivate action.

Older Adults and the 2009 Health and Wellness Segmentation Study

Older adults (defined in this case as the 50–64, 65–74, and ≥ 75 years age groups) comprised 62 percent of the *I Need a Plan* segment identified in the 2009 Health and Wellness Segmentation Study. They need to be provided with checklists and guidance, and they need to be held accountable so that they are more fully engaged. With respect to providing guidance, Bodhaine remarked that many consumers (in all segments, not just *I Need a Plan*) turn to four or five sources of information before making decisions about health. Much of this information is on the Internet. Yet when people go online, they tend to be "absolutely confused" by what they read. Creating harmony among these multiple sources of information is a challenge. Bodhaine stressed the importance of consolidating this information into something meaningful and credible.

Fortunately, older adults comprise 54 percent of the *Leading the Way* segment, but this segment comprises only 10 percent of the U.S. population. Nonetheless, people in this group can be evangelical in their ability to help others make changes.

In general, older adults tend to be more serious about their health than younger adults and do everything they can to remain well. For example, according to 2009 Health and Wellness Segmentation Study data, 75 percent of adults age 65 and over reported having a physical within the past year, compared to 55 percent of the total study population. Also, 53 percent of adults age 65 and over agreed with the statement, "I am very focused on my long-term health and work hard to make decisions every day that will positively influence my future and health and wellness," compared to 44 percent of the total study population. Many younger adults think that health is important but have other priorities. Also, many younger adults believe that they have the power to change their health behaviors but they do not have the attention span—they have higher priorities. Bodhaine said that as people get older and no longer have the pressure of work and other elements, they have time to focus more on health.

Emotion plays a large part in how older consumers think about health. People with four or five chronic conditions often report that their health is good, and they consider themselves healthy because they have a positive outlook on life, wonderful family relationships, and a sense of purpose. The emotion of wellness can mask the physical reality of disease. Bodhaine stated that in order to motivate health behavior change in older adults, these other tenets of wellness must be embraced and couched within a broader, holistic view of health. For example, the need to be part of a community and feel a sense of connection as well as the need to stay active mentally and socially are very important drivers of perceived well-being and, therefore, health.

Health 3.0

Bodhaine repeated that single messages do not work and that communication must be personally relevant. He introduced the concepts of Health 1.0, Health 2.0, and Health 3.0. Health 1.0 is physician-centered (i.e., the "Marcus Welby, MD, doctor-knows-best environment"), Health 2.0 is consumer-centric health care, and Health 3.0 is the new era of accountability. Health 2.0 is not working because "consumers cannot get there alone." Many consumers have neither the education nor experience to use BMI calculators and other tools. Now, with Health 3.0, individuals are held personally accountable for health behavior change, driven largely by workplace wellness initiatives. For example, North Carolina introduced a new program to begin in 2011 whereby overweight or obese individuals will pay a premium for their health insurance. Bodhaine concluded by stating, "The age of accountability has come. How can we harness that in a positive, productive way to really motivate behavior change?"

FOOD SAFETY MESSAGES: WHAT DO CONSUMERS HEAR?

Presenter: Caroline Smith DeWaal

DeWaal began by remarking that the Center for Science in the Public Interest (CSPI) is a binational consumer advocacy organization founded in 1971 by Michael Jacobson. CSPI has been communicating with consumers for nearly four decades, with a focus on nutrition, health, and food safety. In addition to their *Nutrition Action Healthletter*, CSPI maintains an outbreak database and publishes an annual *Outbreak Alert!* Report. The center represents 950,000 subscribers/members in the United States and Canada. She said that her talk would address not just whether CSPI, but also government, is effectively communicating about food safety with the public. She identified two underlying themes of her talk: (1) Government itself needs communication education. Many government messages and tools "are not yet hitting the mark." Government programs need to develop greater expertise in handling risk communication in a way that elicits the appropriate consumer response. (2) A key lesson learned from past outbreaks is that while people do not always take steps to protect themselves, they will take steps to protect people they care about. She said, "Sometimes if you aim for a different mark, you hit your target." As such, targeting messages to families of elderly consumers is often helpful.

Risk Communication with Older Adults

Risk communication with older adults is especially important because older adults are at greater risk for severe illness and death from unsafe food. FoodNet[1] data from 2009 show that, among laboratory-isolated cases of illness from *Listeria* and Shiga toxin-producing *E. Coli* (STEC) O157, the majority of hospitalizations occurred among adults age 50 and over (Vugia et. al., 2009) (see Table 6-1). A large percentage of hospitalizations for illnesses from other pathogens was also among adults 50 years and older. Further, the case fatality rate was highest in the 50 and over population for several pathogens (see Table 6-2).

DeWaal noted several general observations about older adult consumers that should be kept in mind when considering how best to deliver urgent messages.

TABLE 6-1 Percentage of Hospitalizations Composed of Adults Aged 50 or Over

Pathogen	Percent of Hospitalizations
Listeria	86
STEC O157	53
Vibrio	45
Salmonella	40
Yersinia	38
Shigella	28
Cryptosporidium	25
Campylobacter	21

SOURCE: Vugia et al., 2009.

TABLE 6-2 Fatality Rate of Foodborne Illness in Adults Aged 50 or Over

Pathogen	Percent of Fatalities
Listeria	20
Vibrio	7
Salmonella	1.3
Shigella	0.4
Campylobacter	0.4

SOURCE: Vugia et al., 2009.

[1] For additional discussion about CDC FoodNet data, see the summary of Steven Gendel's presentation in Chapter 4.

Older consumers

- Listen to radio and TV regularly. In fact, most consumers of all ages get food recall information from radio or TV.
- Are willing to follow label directions (e.g., "For safety, freeze or discard after January 14.").
- May not be technologically "savvy." DeWaal said that the elderly may be the fastest-growing segment of Internet users (as Bodhaine had remarked), and future elderly populations may rely on the Internet for information, but it is highly unlikely that the Internet will become a major source of information for the current elderly population.
- May not be current with newspapers.
- May be less willing to throw away food.

Case Examples of Communication Challenges

DeWaal discussed several case examples illustrating the communication challenges of food safety recalls:

- *The Peanut Corporation of America (PCA) recall*: The 2009 PCA *Salmonella typhimurium* outbreak sickened hundreds of people and killed nine. It was a very serious outbreak that demanded urgent risk communication. The government implemented three novel communication technologies as part of its recall strategy, none of which were very effective: (1) The Food and Drug Administration's (FDA's) Peanut Product Recall Widget, which was useful to some people but too technological for the elderly and other vulnerable groups. (2) FDA on Twitter, which is out of the realm of experience of many elderly and other vulnerable groups. (3) An online spreadsheet with line listings of recalled products, which was very difficult for consumers to use.
- *Honduran cantaloupes recall*: In response to the 2008 cantaloupe *Salmonella* outbreak, FDA put out a press release stating, "The cantaloupes were distributed for sale . . . in cardboard cartons with the brand 'Dole' and 'PRODUCT OF HONDURAS' printed on each of the side panels of the carton." The problem with this, DeWaal said, is that consumers, especially older consumers, do not buy cantaloupes by the carton. It was impossible for consumers to know whether the single cantaloupe they had just purchased was part of the recall. Now, there is a country-of-origin label requirement, but it is unclear how far this label will go and if, for example, half, sliced, or cut-up cantaloupes will be required to have the label.

- *Hallmark/Westland Meat Packing Co. beef recall*: The recall notice from the U.S. Department of Agriculture (USDA) for the 2008 beef recall read, "Hallmark/Westland Meat Packing Co . . . is voluntarily recalling approximately 143,383,823 pounds of raw and frozen beef products that FSIS (Food Safety and Inspection Service) has determined to be unfit for human food because the cattle did not receive complete and proper inspection." The problem here was that most consumers do not know what a "voluntary" recall is. While it is technically accurate that all food recalls other than infant formula recalls are voluntary, most consumers interpret use of the word "voluntary" to mean that the recall is not serious. Otherwise, the recall would be mandatory. DeWaal stated that use of the word "voluntary" is counterproductive and paradoxical; how can something that the government has deemed unfit for human consumption be only voluntarily recalled? Since this press release was issued, USDA has changed its policy.

DeWaal said that, in general, much of the recall information posted online by FDA and USDA is not useful to the public. For example, neither agency has a searchable database (i.e., consumers cannot search by commodity, data, pathogen, brand name, etc.). DeWaal mentioned the combined FDA/USDA information site, www.foodsafety.gov, and said she expects that it will be an improvement. In comparison, several nongovernmental organizations have stepped in to provide needed information. CSPI has an Outbreak Alert webpage (http://www.cspinet.org/foodsafety) where consumers can search for recall information and a database that allows consumers to review historical outbreak information by food, pathogen, or state. Safe Tables Our Priority also sends daily e-mail alerts notifying the public of pending outbreaks and recalls.

Direct-to-Consumer Notification

DeWaal identified direct-to-consumer notification as a potentially good strategy for reaching older consumers with urgent food safety messages. In particular CSPI is recommending the following:

- Retailers should use loyalty programs to notify consumers of Class I recalls (the most serious category of recalls, involving a potential for serious injury or death). For example, Costco did this during the PCA outbreak, notifying more than 1.5 million consumers by phone and many more by mail that they had purchased a product that was the subject of a Class I recall. This was a very important and effective way of reaching their customers.

- Recall notifications should be posted at retail stores and on shelves where recalled products were sold. DeWaal emphasized that this type of on-the-spot communicating does not mean posting a notice on a bulletin board near the entrance to the store, where consumers rarely stop, but rather right on the shelf near the product being sold. Shoppers tend to be "creatures of habit," going back to the same aisles and shelves to retrieve the same product they bought last week. This type of on-the-spot information would be very effective in terms of alerting customers to problems in products they have already purchased.

Food Safety in Restaurants

While the food industry often claims that food safety problems are the responsibility of consumers, data indicate that between 1999 and 2006, 41 percent of 5,778 outbreaks in the United States were sourced to foods prepared in restaurants or food establishments (Figure 6-1). Targeting restaurant food safety is a very important but often overlooked need.

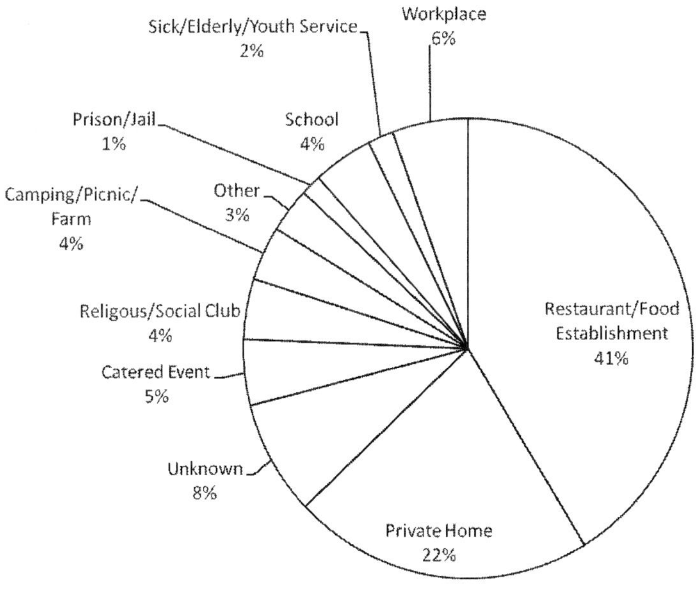

FIGURE 6-1 Outbreaks of food safety problems by location, 1999–2006 (n = 5,778).
SOURCE: CSPI, Outbreak Alert! Database, 2008.

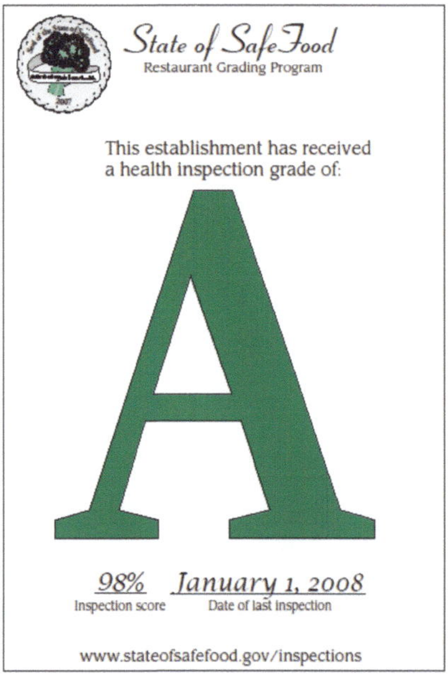
State of Safe Food
Restaurant Grading Program
This establishment has received
a health inspection grade of:
A
98%
Inspection score
January 1, 2008
Date of last inspection
www.stateofsafefood.gov/inspections

FIGURE 6-2 Example of a letter grade sign that would be displayed in the window of a food establishment.
SOURCE: CSPI, 2008.

In 2008, CSPI released the *Dirty Dining* report comparing restaurant inspections in twenty U.S. cities. The report was based on inspection reports from local health departments; it rated both transparency (i.e., how easy it is for consumers to obtain inspection information in order to make a choice about where to eat) and inspection effectiveness (i.e., what the inspections revealed). In the report, CSPI recommends that every city adopt a letter grade system, similar to the system Los Angeles County uses, and which has proven effective there. The L.A. restaurant industry overall has improved since the letter grade system was adopted, because having any grade but an "A" posted in the front window is considered a disgrace. An example of letter grade signage is shown in Figure 6-2. DeWaal stated that L.A. County documented reductions in foodborne illness and emergency room visits following initiation of the letter grade system.

Letter grades are really just another form of on-the-spot messaging. Consumers are information seekers, but they are also busy and want the information when they need it. DeWaal said that while the letter grade is proving effective, the program could become even stronger by making the actual and complete results of the restaurant inspections readily available to consumers (e.g., on the Internet).

Conclusion

In conclusion, DeWaal stated that food safety communication cannot rely on the Internet alone. This is particularly true with respect to recalls. Most consumers, not just the elderly population, hear about recalls from radio or TV. She said that on-the-spot messaging must be more seriously considered as an additional way to communicate urgent food safety messages.

COMMUNICATING WITH OLDER CONSUMERS DURING RECALLS

Presenter: William Hallman

Hallman began by remarking that his research at the Food Policy Institute (FPI) at Rutgers University[2] was funded by USDA Cooperative State Research, Education, and Extension Service through the National Integrated Food Safety Initiative and was designed to address issues related to intentional and unintentional food contamination. The project started with the question, "How do we help consumers regain confidence in the food supply after an incident of food contamination?" Given that there was virtually no academic literature concerning how consumers deal with food recalls, one of FPI's first actions was to develop a survey aimed at gaining a better understanding of what consumers know and do when recalls occur. While assembling the survey, the *E. coli* O157 spinach outbreak (September 2006) occurred. FPI researchers took advantage of this "natural experiment" and surveyed what people heard, knew, and did in response to the spinach outbreak. They also conducted key informant interviews with public and industry officials and analyzed FDA and industry press releases and media coverage. The results of the survey, *Public Response to the Contaminated Spinach Recall of 2006*, are available online at www.foodpolicy.rutgers.edu.

The *Public Response to the Contaminated Spinach Recall of 2006* survey led to collaboration with the Grocery Manufacturers Association (GMA), whereby GMA funded a national survey on public perceptions of food recalls in general. FPI also conducted an associated analysis of TV and newspaper coverage of food recalls. Coincidentally, while as-

[2] FPI was founded in 1999 as a Board of Governors Research Institute at Rutgers University, with the mission of addressing key issues in the production, marketing, distribution, sales, consumption, and regulation of food and other agricultural products. As an academic research institute, its role is to provide unbiased information and education that is timely, relevant, and responsive to the needs of government, industry, and the consumer.

sembling this survey and analysis, the *Salmonella* Saintpaul outbreak in tomatoes occurred, and so again, FPI took advantage of a "natural experiment" and examined what Americans heard, knew, and did in response to the *Salmonella* Saintpaul recall. The results of both the general survey (*Consumer Responses to Food Recalls: 2008 National Survey Report*) and the "natural experiment" (*Public Response to the* Salmonella *Saintpaul Outbreak of 2008*) are also available online at www.foodpolicy.rutgers.edu.

The Need for Better Recall Communication

Hallman briefly discussed the "realities" of the food supply and food recalls. The supply and demand for agricultural products is becoming increasingly global, while food processing, distribution, and retail are becoming increasingly consolidated. As a result, there is increasing competition to supply commodities year-round and at the lowest prices. The end result is increasing complexity in the supply chain, potentially increased anonymity in the overall system (i.e., as it becomes more complex), and different quality and safety standards among different cultures, countries, and regions.

At the same time, both the Centers for Disease Control and Prevention (CDC) and state health departments have strengthened their abilities to identify patterns of foodborne illness through the use of improved epidemiological surveillance systems and enhanced analytical capabilities. For example, "DNA fingerprint" technology now allows for the identification of particular strains of outbreak pathogens, and other technologies have the capacity to more rapidly detect contaminants, and in increasingly smaller amounts. These breakthroughs have made it easier to identify foodborne illness outbreaks which often lead to food recalls. Hallman said that in the future, as these technologies continue to improve, the number of food recalls will likely increase. Therefore, it is essential that food recall communications improve.

"Getting it right" (i.e., getting better at communicating about food recalls) means alerting the public, motivating the public to take appropriate actions in response to the problem, ceasing such actions after the problem has been resolved, and not creating unnecessary fright or loss of confidence in the food supply throughout the process. "Getting it wrong" means unnecessary illnesses and deaths because the public does not hear the message or does not take appropriate action; unnecessary avoidance of healthful, nutritious foods because the public is frightened; companies going bankrupt; and consumers losing confidence in the food system.

Echoing some of DeWaal's remarks, Hallman emphasized that communicating about food recalls with older adults is particularly important because older consumers are especially vulnerable to serious illness or death resulting from exposure to foodborne pathogens. Older adults are also more likely than younger adults to prepare and eat meals at home and to have poor food safety practices that can increase the risk of infection (e.g., the literature suggests that many older adults have refrigerators or freezers that are too warm, are reluctant to discard products after expired "use-by-dates," and increasingly rely on smell or taste to determine wholesomeness). Plus, older consumers are increasingly reliant on "heat-and-serve," "ready-to-eat," and other prepared convenience products. Many consumers automatically think that a food product wrapped in plastic is already safe to eat (what Hallman has called the "cellophane effect") or that a package that will fit in the microwave needs only to be heated and served, ignoring the directions, which are often written in tiny script on the back of the box.

Communicating with Older Adults: The Problem of Invisibility

Improving communication about food recalls with older adults in particular is also important because of the invisibility of foodborne pathogens. Because such pathogens cannot be seen, consumers must rely on other cues, mostly visual and olfactory cues, to determine whether something is safe to eat. Without those cues, it is easy for people to ignore or amplify the real risks. When consumers cannot verify safety for themselves, they have to trust others to tell them what is safe to eat. As an example of the challenge associated with knowing whether something is potentially contaminated with an invisible pathogen, Hallman showed a picture of a bag of pistachios with a corner of the bag missing. He had purchased the nuts himself and had already opened the bag when the grocery store where he had purchased them called him to notify him of a pistachio recall due to potential contamination with *Salmonella*. He said that he would otherwise never have known about the risk, despite being "in the business."

Another problem with invisibility, he said, is that consumers have difficulty distinguishing which products are included in recalls. Interpretable information (e.g., lot or batch number, "sell by date") is often not readily identifiable. Labels containing that type of information can be difficult to locate or read even for consumers without vision problems, and many manufacturers' code numbers have no meaning for consumers. Moreover, many fresh produce items lack such information altogether. In the 2008 survey that FPI conducted in collaboration with GMA, only 13 percent of respondents who looked for a recalled food product said that they used such information to tell whether the product had been recalled (Hallman et al., 2009). Some people adopt a "better safe than sorry" strategy, with 28 percent of respondents saying that they had simply thrown out food in response to a recall. Others avoid products that are similar to those that have been recalled or that were made by the same company. Some companies try to do the distinguishing themselves. Hallman showed an image of a manufacturer's shelf label in a store indicating that their brand of peanut butter was "not part of the peanut recall."

Hallman emphasized the importance of providing consumers with a means to easily identify affected and unaffected products. This should include providing specific information, such as lot numbers and product dates that will help consumers clearly differentiate between safe and potentially unsafe products.

Misconceptions and Reactions to Food Recalls

Many people know very little about foodborne illness, including how to recognize symptoms. Often, people confuse foodborne illness with the mythical "24-hour flu." Many people do not realize that symptoms of common foodborne illnesses may not appear until several days after ingestion, and they often blame the last thing they ate. Many also do not seem to recognize that some foodborne pathogens can have more serious consequences than others. Finally, people make little distinction between particular contaminants—they are more concerned with the fact that something is contaminated than they are with the pathogen itself. Hallman emphasized the importance of educating people about symptoms, not just about the number of illnesses and deaths (a more detailed discussion about the type of details media coverage usually includes is to follow).

Similarly, many people know very little about food recalls. In one FPI survey, 73 percent of Americans indicated that FDA is responsible for meat and poultry recalls, when in fact USDA is the responsible authority (Hallman et al., 2009). Also, 80 percent of respondents indicated that under U.S. law, the government can force any food company to recall a contaminated product, when in fact it cannot. People also underestimate the number of food recalls. Hallman said that part of the challenge is language. For example, there are three classes of recalls (I, II, and III) with corresponding levels of severity of the potential consequences of consuming the contaminated product, but those categories mean nothing to consumers. Many people do not even know when a recall is occurring and are confused by the terms "advisory" and "voluntary recalls." Hallman added that while under current regulations, regardless of the severity of the contamination problem, all recalls of food products (except for baby formula) are technically "voluntary." However, since most consumers believe the government has the power to compel companies to recall contaminated products, the public may believe that if a food product is recalled voluntarily, the reason for the recall may not be very serious.

However, people do pay attention to high profile recalls. In FPI surveys, 87 percent of respondents heard about the 2006 spinach recall (Cuite et al., 2007), 93 percent had heard about the 2008 tomato recall, and 68 percent had heard about the 2008 pepper recall (Cuite et al., 2008). When asked if a certain product had been recalled within the last two years, 81 percent said yes to ground beef, but only 23 percent said yes to canned chili (and that product had been recalled within six to eight months of the survey), and only 17 percent said yes to cantaloupe (Hallman et al., 2009). When asked if they had heard about a recall of raw potatoes, which in fact never happened, 8 percent said yes. Hallman noted that the last result highlights the fact that people are subject to social desirability biases and will "tell you what they think you want to hear." The social psychological literature suggests that older consumers are even more subject to this particular bias. He cautioned that one must interpret survey data "with a grain of salt."

FPI survey data indicate that most Americans first hear about recalls from TV, which is how 71 percent of respondents first heard about the 2006 spinach recall (the remainder heard about it from the radio [9 percent], other people [8 percent], newspapers [5 percent], and "other" [7 percent]) and how 66 percent first heard about the 2008 tomato recall (the remainder heard about it from the radio [9 percent], restaurants [6 percent], stores [2 percent], and "other" [17 percent]) (Cuite et al., 2007, 2008). Hallman reiterated what previous speakers had stated about patterns of media use varying by age and that while younger older Americans (i.e., people younger than 55) are accessing the Internet, adults 55 and older still rely primarily on newspapers and both national and local TV news.

FPI's analyses of TV and newspaper coverage during the spinach recall and tomato/pepper warnings indicate that coverage in the news about "what to do" is often lacking (Nucci et al., 2009). The focus tends to be on the number of deaths and illnesses and on the progress of the investigation. There is usually very little focus on which products are safe to eat, details concerning what is unsafe, symptoms of illness, groups of people particularly at risk (e.g., elderly or immunocompromised individuals), and practical information about how to avoid becoming ill. Hallman emphasized the need to educate people about what to do in response to a recall.

In addition to getting information from the media, many people get information from other people. According to one FPI survey, 84 percent of respondents said they talked about the 2006 spinach recall with others, and 30 percent said they did so occasionally or frequently (Cuite et al., 2007). The problem with this is that people do not always get the information right. For example, while almost everybody knew that bags of fresh spinach had been recalled (95 percent), a significant number of people also thought (incorrectly) that frozen (22 percent) and canned spinach (16 percent) had been recalled as well. During the *Salmonella* Saintpaul incident, only 31 percent of respondents strongly agreed that they knew which types of tomatoes the public had been warned not to eat (Cuite et al., 2008).

FPI survey data also indicate that people generalize to other foods in response to recalls. During the spinach outbreak, 18 percent of respondents who had heard about the recall stopped eating other bagged produce, including lettuce and other ingredients (Cuite et al., 2007). Forty-eight percent said that they washed their produce more thoroughly as a result of the recall, even though this was not recommended as a way to make spinach safe. There were no differences between spinach eaters and non-eaters in these behaviors. Hallman emphasized the importance of sending specific messages and repeating information about what is safe versus unsafe.

FPI survey data also suggest that people conduct personal risk assessments when they hear recall information. In a GMA-sponsored study, participants were asked how important they think it is for news stories to include information about various aspects of a food recall (Table 6-3) (Hallman et al., 2009). Interestingly, "the illnesses and symptoms caused by eating the recalled product" was at the top of the list, with a mean score of 92 (with 0 = not at all important and 100 = extremely important), closely followed by "whether anyone has become ill from eating the product" (91), "the date on the package" (91), "the brands affected" (91), and "the lot number on the package" (90). When asked what they would want to know when first hearing about a food recall, 36 percent said identifying information, 21 percent said where the product is from, and 16 percent said where the product is sold/if the person bought some. Together, these data suggest that consumers are trying to assess whether they personally are at risk.

TABLE 6-3 Consumer Survey Responses to the Question, "*How important do you think it is for news stories to include information about . . .*"

	Mean
The illnesses and symptoms caused by eating the recalled product	92
Whether anyone has become ill from eating the product	91
The date on the package	91
The brands affected	91
The lot number on the package	90
What people should do with the product if they find it	88
What is being done to fix the problem that led to the recall	88
The name of the specific contaminant	87
Whether anything can be done to make the product safe to eat, such as cooking it	84
How the contamination happened	82

SOURCE: Food Policy Institute, 2009 (Hallman et al., 2009).

Hallman stated that the problem with conducting personal risk assessments is that some people are predisposed to believing they are not at risk. For example, when asked what food they buy often is most likely to be subject to a recall, 50 percent of respondents said a meat product; 22 percent said produce; 9 percent said fish, dairy, or other; and only 19 percent said they did not know (Hallman et al., 2009). When asked how likely the food they purchased will be recalled compared to other Americans purchasing the same food product, 38 percent said "somewhat less" or "much less." Hallman described these results as "classic optimistic bias." While people believe that food recalls are important, some do not believe that recalls necessarily apply to them. This kind of "unrealistic optimism" has been observed in connection with many kinds of health behaviors.

In fact, Hallman stated, "the default position for most consumers is apathy." In one FPI survey, only 59 percent of respondents said that they had ever looked for a recalled product in their home, and only 10 percent said they had found a recalled product in their home (Hallman et al., 2009). Although most people hear about large recalls, few people are actually motivated to look for the recalled products in their homes. While some behaviors show no age-related differences (e.g., whether a consumer checks their home for the recalled product and whether he or she found a recalled product), people below the age of 55 were more likely than people over age 55 to have eaten a food that they knew had been recalled. When people do not think that recalls apply to them, they do not take action.

Getting It Right

Hallman discussed two ways that recall communication could be improved: (1) using personalized messaging and (2) making specific calls to action.

Personalized Messaging

As prior speakers had done, Hallman emphasized that consumers would like more personalized messages about food recalls. FPI survey data show that about three-quarters of Americans (all ages) would like such information as part of receipts at the grocery store. In other words, they would like point-of-purchase information, which Hallman stated is an excellent way to communicate information to consumers and to convince them that the recall applies to them. Some companies are beginning to use grocery store "loyalty card" information to contact their customers when they have purchased a product that is later recalled and consumers seem receptive to the practice. He predicts that in the future there be will more personalized communications related to food and other types of recalls.

He also emphasized there is no single "public" and that there are multiple audiences with varying knowledge, experiences, and attitudes. Market segmentation and tailored recall messages are an important means of communicating in a way that motivates consumers to respond appropriately.

Making Specific Calls to Action

Hallman also emphasized the importance of specific calls to action. After judging that they are at risk, consumers want to know how to reduce that risk. For example, should they throw out the product, or can they wash and cook it? Some people, however, do not follow advice. For example, during the *Salmonella* Saintpaul outbreak, 93 percent of survey respondents said that they had heard about the warning not to eat tomatoes (Cuite et al., 2008). Of those 93 percent, 80 percent said they had eaten tomatoes before the warning. Of those 80 percent, 64 percent said they had eaten tomatoes during the warning. Of those, 36 percent ate tomatoes that were included in the warning. Of those, 89 percent were aware of the warning at the moment they ate the tomatoes. When asked why they ate tomatoes that were considered not safe (Table 6-4), 41 percent said "I thought they wouldn't hurt me"; 13 percent said "I distrust the government and/or media"; 13 percent said "It must be safe if it's being sold"; and 12 percent said "I made it safe (e.g., washed it, cooked it)." Thus some people knowingly eat recalled foods. Overall, according to FPI data, about 12 percent of Americans have eaten a food that they thought had been recalled. Hallman expressed concern that the lack of apparent consequences is likely to weaken confidence in future warnings.

TABLE 6-4 Survey Respondents' Reasons for Eating Recalled Tomatoes

Statement	Percentage Citing
I thought they wouldn't hurt me	41
I distrust the government and/or media	13
It must be safe if it is being sold	13
I made it safe (e.g., washed it, cooked it)	12
Other	20

NOTE: n = 124; statements were responses to the question, "Why did you eat the tomatoes that were considered safe not to eat?"
SOURCE: Food Policy Institute, 2008 (Cuite et al., 2008).

Unlike many other health-related messages about food, recalls are generally limited in scope and time. But even "all-clear" messages (i.e., that the food is safe to eat again) are not getting through. A week and a half after lifting the tomato advisory, only 46 percent of respondents aware of the advisory "strongly agreed" that authorities considered it okay to eat tomatoes again (Cuite et al., 2008). Six weeks after the end of the 2006 spinach recall, only 55 percent of respondents who were aware of the recall thought it was "definitely true" that authorities said that spinach available in supermarkets was safe to eat (Cuite et al., 2007). Hallman emphasized the importance of reassuring consumers that the problem that led to the recall has been fixed and that it is safe to eat the product again. Both industry and government need to work on messages that reinforce this.

Conclusion

In conclusion, Hallman restated what he had said at the beginning of his talk: improvements in foodborne illness outbreak surveillance and the ability to identify outbreak strains of pathogens are likely to lead to more warnings, advisories, market withdrawals, and recalls in the future. Therefore, getting the communication right is essential.

COMMUNICATING NUTRITION MESSAGES TO OLDER PERSONS

Presenter: Ronni Chernoff

Chernoff began by noting that the Arkansas Geriatric Education Center addresses health literacy but does not deal directly with consumers, rather it deals with the people who deal with consumers. She listed a number of key findings from the National Assessment of Adult Literacy, which measures American adults' literacy skills.[3]

- Adults age 65 and over have lower health literacy scores than any other age group. In general, older adults tend to be less educated than the rest of the population.
- Women have higher literacy scores than men. Chernoff explained that this is probably because women tend to pay more attention to health messages, because they are the primary caregivers for their children as well as for their older parents.

---

[3] National Center for Education Statistics, 2003.

- Adults with low literacy are more likely to get health information from radio and television than from written sources.
- Adults with higher literacy receive their health information from newspapers, magazines, books, brochures, or the Internet. Chernoff mentioned how difficult it has been to conduct online courses and reach a point where even health professionals in rural areas are taking part, making the idea of getting consumers to use the Internet for accessing health information seem even more challenging.

For the remainder of her presentation, Chernoff discussed the elements of effective written and oral communication. She stressed the importance of reinforcing key messages, for example by giving consumers something to take home after the interaction. Often, most of what has been said is forgotten by the time people walk out the door. Giving them something to take home reinforces key messages.

The Elements of Effective Written Communication

First, she listed and described elements of effective written communication:

- *Develop easy-to-read forms.* Health professionals often feel the need to communicate so much information that they develop complicated forms that people with low literacy levels may have difficulty understanding.
- *Use plain language.* Health professionals often feel the need to impress people by using "big words," which may be self-gratifying but not helpful.
- *Provide relevant examples.* Reiterating comments from previous speakers, Chernoff emphasized the importance of making communication personal and providing examples of how information is likely to affect the consumer.
- *Be specific.* Talking in global terms does not help people understand how information might potentially affect them.
- *Get client to give feedback by asking questions.* Asking the client to reflect what they heard increases the likelihood that the message is understood.
- *Provide forms in many languages.* America is a country of increasingly diverse languages.
- *Train staff to provide assistance.* It is important that all staff be able to assist people in interpreting the information that has been provided.
- *Limit messages to a few key points.* Providing a large amount of information can easily overwhelm. By "keeping it simple," messages are more likely to be internalized.

- *Present concrete examples.* Providing concrete examples gives people an "anchor" that helps them hold onto the information.
- *Repeat and reinforce the most important points.*
- *Provide culturally appropriate and age appropriate content.* People must be able to fit information into what they know based on their life experiences. Chernoff mentioned that some of the geriatric education centers in Oklahoma, for example, deal with many Native Americans and therefore must communicate information in a way that fits into an experience that is very different than that of other Americans.
- *Ensure the reading level is no higher than 5th grade, or 3rd grade for limited literacy groups.* This is challenging for professionals who are accustomed to writing for and speaking to professional audiences, but it is the only way to reach many consumers. Chernoff mentioned how easy it is for consumers to confuse *Listeria* with *Wisteria*, for example, or to think that *Listeria* has something to do with Listerine. Many consumers have no framework for the word "*Listeria*"; they don't know what it is or how to process the information.
- *Add simple drawings to explain what you are talking about.*
- *Avoid too much detail and complex diagrams.* Diagrams with too many lines and colors end up having very little meaning for most people.
- *Provide visual step-by-step diagrams or pictures.* For example, to illustrate how to give an insulin injection or how to take pills.
- *Use large type font (at least 12 point).* Many older adults cannot read small print, even with glasses or after surgery.
- *Limit number of fonts.* Fancy or varying fonts can be visually exhausting, particularly for older adults.
- *Avoid all capital letters.* ALL CAPS tend to run together, making them difficult to read.
- *Use headings and bullets.* Headings and bullets can be helpful in organizing information in a logical, rational way.
- *Avoid long sentences.* Again, try to maintain a 5th grade reading level.
- *Leave white space.* Too much information on a page and small margins can turn readers away.
- *Use strong contrast colors.* Chernoff remarked that initially, she and her colleagues assumed that older adults would want information presented in pastel colors (e.g., light yellows, pinks, and blues). But they discovered that older adults prefer strong colors because of the contrast, which makes reading easier.
- *Use captions to highlight information.* Highlighting information is a way to reinforce key messages.

The Elements of Effective Oral Communication

Chernoff then listed and described elements of effective oral communication:

- *Listen.* Chernoff called listening "perhaps the single most important thing in oral communication."
- *Speak slowly.* When speaking with older adults or to somebody for whom English is not the primary language, it is important not to yell but rather to speak slowly.
- *Sit during the meeting.* Being face-to-face and not looking down on someone is less intimidating for them.
- *Have the individal respond to what you have said.* Getting feedback is the only way to know whether somebody understands the information.
- *Encourage questions.* Ask, "What questions do you have?" and not "Do you have any questions?" When asked the latter, most people will respond "no." Encouraging clients to ask specific questions is more effective.
- *Use plain language.*
- *Create an opportunity for dialogue or conversation.*
- *Create orienting statements* (e.g., "First let's talk about your favorite food . . ."). For example, asking somebody to talk about a favorite food is a better way to initiate conversation than asking if they eat vegetables.
- *Limit information at each meeting.*
- *Stress the most important point* (e.g., "Your blood sugar is too high and we need to discuss what you can do to control it.").
- *Review the most important point.*
- *Draw or use pictures to illustrate a point.*
- *Use verbal and written explanation together, not just one or the other.*
- *Verify understanding of material.*
- *Summarize the meeting and conclude by telling the individual what to expect next.*
- *Keep sessions brief and focus on one point.* Chernoff said that, based on her experience, it is unlikely that people who have been eating a certain way for 75 years are going to change their entire diet. Focusing on one thing rather than their overall diet stands a better chance of motivating change.
- *Relate new information to past experience.* Use stories or personal examples.

- *Present information one step at a time and omit unnecessary information.*
- *Create a supportive environment.* Have an attitude of helpfulness; create a quiet place; have straight-backed chairs; use large and easy-to-follow signs; and assist with follow-up scheduling.
- *Use engaging methods* (e.g., video examples or take-home materials with telephone numbers).

QUESTIONS AND DISCUSSION

The four presentations prompted many questions from the audience about recalls, the concept of opt-out strategizing, the concept of persuading by reason but motivating through emotion, the use of symbols to convey food safety information, and the challenge of sending simple messages about complicated situations.

Food Recalls

Several questions on food recalls initiated a discussion that compared food recalls to recalls of other consumer goods and the possibilities for enhancing food recall communication.

Compliance with Food Recalls

Hallman was asked how compliance with food recalls compares with recalls for other types of products. Hallman said that he did not know but that part of the problem with food recalls is that often by the time the food is recalled, it is either past its shelf life or the majority has already been consumed. Often it is difficult to find a recalled food item in the home. It is easier to find recalled tires, for example, and therefore compliance with a recall of that type of non-food item might be higher.

Improving Food Recall Communication

All of the presenters were asked to provide their opinions on what could be done to improve food recall communication. DeWaal emphasized the importance of reminding consumers that something they had purchased was being recalled. Retail notification would be a very direct way to send this reminder. Additionally, information should be posted on stores shelves where the product is located, notifying shoppers of the recall and requesting that they please return the product. She also mentioned that most government food recall communications are targeted at retailers, not the consuming public, even though they are published for the public. For example, during the 2008 Honduran cantaloupe recall, while it was important to communicate with retailers, it would also have been very helpful for consumers to know whether the single cantaloupe they had purchased was part of the recall.

Groth suggested placing coupon dispensers with information about food recalls in aisles, instead of or in addition to information on the shelves. That way, people could take coupons containing all of the necessary information about the recalled product (e.g., brand, lot number) and see if they actually have any recalled product in their home.

Bodhaine said that it is important to repeatedly deliver an accurate message through a credible channel. He said that consumers usually have to hear a message seven times before they realize that it pertains to them. He said that a local voice is more credible to consumers than a distant voice. For example, local stores may be more credible than Congress. Also, given that consumers are turning to multiple sources of information "in search of the truth," it is important that the same message be delivered across all platforms (e.g., physicians, WebMD, and MayoClinic.com[4]). Bodhaine also emphasized the importance of telling consumers not just what to do but why they should be doing it.

Chernoff stated that sending the same message through multiple media is very important, because people do not necessarily receive messages from the same sources. She emphasized the importance of "keeping it simple," "keeping it repetitive," and "having it accessible in multiple ways."

Hallman emphasized the importance of reinforcing the message that older consumers really need to pay attention to the issue at hand. Through such reinforcement, even if the older consumers themselves do not hear the message, their children and friends may. For example, one reason influenza vaccinations in older adults have a fairly high compliance rate is because many children nudge their parents to "go do this." Hallman also emphasized the need for a searchable database where food recall information can be easily accessed, for example some kind of tool that allows consumers to scan a food bar code to see if that particular food product has been recalled. He mentioned the 2009 PCA recall and the large number of consumers that refused to buy any peanut butter products, even those not affected by the recall, because they were afraid. Having some sort of application, for example on smart phones, whereby consumers could simply scan the barcode and see whether in fact the product in hand was on a recall list would alleviate some of this fear.

---

[4] Available online at webmd.com and www.mayoclinic.com/health/DiseasesIndex/DiseasesIndex.

Opt-Out Strategizing

Bodhaine was asked to elaborate on opt-out health solutions. Bodhaine used 401(k) plans as an example. 401(k) retirement plans used to be opt-in, whereby employees had to choose to participate and make a conscientious decision to part with a portion of their income. As a result, enrollments were relatively low and disappointing; so employers began experimenting with the notion of automatically enrolling employees in their 401(k) plans and forcing employees to make a conscientious decision to *not* participate. As a result, enrollments levels increased significantly. In health care, most actions require that consumers make conscientious decisions "to do the right thing in a world that craves convenience." As Bodhaine mentioned during his presentation, "one of the reasons that health is so hard is because life has become so extraordinarily easy." Opt-out health solutions make it easy for consumers to "make the right decision." An example of an opt-out health solution is putting larger labels on fruits and vegetables than on other food items in cafeterias and changing the placement of foods at the check-out counter (e.g. moving salty and sweet foods to the back of the cafeteria and placing fruit up front near checkout). It has been demonstrated at the Mayo Clinic that both of these actions increase consumption of fruits and vegetables. Another opt-out health solution is the 100-calorie snack pack, which makes the decision-making process very simple for the consumer by eliminating the need to calculate calories or estimate serving size.

Groth commented on the likelihood that some people will object to opt-out solutions. Groth agreed with Bodhaine that it makes sense to build incentives into the system to make it easier for people to "do the right thing," but he said that some people might consider opt-out solutions to be coercive. For example, he was once a member of a record club where each member received the monthly record unless he or she mailed a card back to the company requesting that the record not be sent. Many consumers have grown up thinking that opt-out programs, like the old record clubs, are coercive. Bodhaine replied that consumers respond better to nudges than they do mandates, and he encouraged Groth (and others) to read the book *Nudge* (Thaler and Sunstein, 2004).

Persuade by Reason, Motivate Through Emotion

An audience member commented on Bodhaine's "persuade by reason, motivate through emotion" phrase and asked Bodhaine to provide some examples of how communicators could link science and emotion. Bodhaine said that he did not want to undervalue the power of science and that scientific facts provide the "substantive platform" and "reason to believe." However, most consumers rarely understand the science or how to apply it to themselves, or they become bored with the facts. He used car purchasing as an example. Telling a potential buyer what antilock brakes are or how they work does not necessarily motivate a car purchase. The functional benefit of those antilock brakes must somehow be linked to what is important to the consumer (e.g., "my loving concern for my family"). On the other hand, telling a person to buy a car because they love their family is construed as "fluff." He said that the old Michelin ads, with images of children and the tag line "because so much is riding on your tires," were a "brilliant way to demonstrate the added value of creating an emotional link to a tire." He suggested that emotion is often best communicated through cue and symbol rather than word.

DeWaal added that emotion is a natural component of the issue of food safety. Media stories that focus on individuals who have fallen ill from eating contaminated food products naturally lend themselves to providing "a level of emotion and a level of connection." Severe foodborne illnesses are random events. They can happen to anyone, and they cross all socioeconomic and partisan lines. Also, victims are rarely silent or hidden. She mentioned how victims rallied after the Jack-in-the-Box *E. coli* O157:H7 outbreak in 1993 and organized Safe Tables Our Priority (S.T.O.P.). So there is a natural connection between the science and emotion with outbreak data, with victims themselves providing the motivation.

Hallman stated that the challenge for FDA and industry when putting together press releases is to lead with emotion, so that the story is picked up by the media, but then follow up with the critical scientific information so that readers (and consumers) know who is at risk, what those at risk can do to minimize their risk, and what the symptoms of illness are.

Using Symbols to Communicate Food Safety Information

An audience member described North Carolina's restaurant inspection scoring system and how the news media has picked up on it (every week, the local new media list restaurants that have received the highest and lowest scores) and then asked whether any of the presenters had any anecdotal- or study-based thoughts on whether this type of "simple messaging" has proven effective for aging consumers. In addition it was asked whether front-of-package nutrition symbols seem to be of help to older adults. DeWaal replied that food safety messaging does not usually rely on things like front-of-package labeling or other glance messages that are being used for nutrition communication because food recall situations are usually urgent and demand action steps. Convincing consumers not to eat a food product because it is potentially contaminated is a terrific challenge, because many people believe that all food is safe. Even when they know something has been recalled, they eat it. Bodhaine agreed that overcoming consumers' cavalier attitudes about food is a major challenge. There is a belief that "because we do it every day, it must be okay for us."

Bodhaine expressed concern about the way that so many different manufacturers and retailers are launching their own independent food labeling and safety information systems. He said that by introducing a multitude of different symbols and signals to the consumer, "We have taught them once again to ignore us." He said that delivering information in a meaningful way is challenging.

A question was asked about how consumers would differentiate between icons/symbols used for different purposes (e.g., one set of symbols for added sugars, fats, etc.; another set for overall healthfulness; another set for recalls or other safety information). DeWaal stated that CSPI does not recommend rating foods for safety by using symbols or icons on packaging. However, there may be packages with limited shelf lives and with risks linked to the amount of time already shelved (e.g., the risk of *Listeria* contamination in processed meat products). These packages could have a red dot, for instance, indicating that the product is "out of date" or a yellow dot indicating "freeze now and use later," and so on. She mentioned that food scientists are researching this type of application.

Chernoff commented on the need to place expiration dates in places that are more readily accessible. She mentioned that expiration dates on the striated caps of peanut butter jars are unreadable. Placing expiration dates on the label instead of on the striation, as well as in large, highlighted font, would be a simple improvement that would make a big difference.

Hallman commented on the gray market for food products and how dollar stores and the like have erased lot numbers or copied over expiration dates. Many older Americans, particularly those who are food insecure, shop at these establishments.

Bodhaine remarked that the author of the symbol is almost as important as the symbol itself. He said that over the past several years, businesses have knowingly delivered a growing number of bad products and services, and consumers have become increasingly skeptical. He said that government and manufacturers are not always the trusted voices and that collaborative efforts are needed to establish a new trusted voice. Groth agreed and stated that neither is the academic voice the answer, because it speaks in jargon. Bodhaine suggested that the commercial and academic sectors work together to build a platform for moving forward and motivating consumers to change their behaviors.

While on the topic of symbols, Hallman highlighted the challenge of using package symbols to communicate microwave instructions, given that different microwaves have different wattages and that microwave times differ dramatically. He mentioned that some retailers are beginning to match symbols on their food packages with symbols on microwaves indicating which microwave button to push in order to thoroughly heat the package in question, but the issue needs to be addressed more fully.

Groth pointed to *Consumer Reports*' iconic five-point quality symbol system (excellent, very good, good, fair, poor) as an example of successfully quantifying in an understandable way a very complicated phenomenon. That system can be used to characterize products based on ratings of 20 or more different properties. He suggested that a similar system might be worth considering for conveying information about food safety.

Sending Simple Messages About Complicated Situations

Groth mentioned that several speakers had emphasized the need to keep messages simple so that they can be understood. However, the situation at hand is often very complicated. For example, FDA's list of foods that older adults should not eat (which Sundlof had described during his presentation in an earlier session) includes raw fish. Groth said that he loves raw fish and eats it several times a week, and that he is more concerned with his long-term cardiovascular health than he is the risk of becoming ill from eating contaminated raw fish. "So I am making risk-risk tradeoffs. In fact, a lot of the world is," he said. "If we oversimplify the message too much, we will steer people into bad behavior. So how do we deal with that?" DeWaal mentioned that outbreak data indicate that sushi is not implicated very often. Groth said that he is worried about the "generic problem," not sushi in particular. DeWaal replied that the generic problem could be with FDA's message. She said, "It is absolutely true that any high-risk consumer should avoid certain raw seafood. . . . It is vital that that message get out. . . . If they are saying avoid all raw seafood, that may be overstating a problem that really is more isolated."

Bodhaine said that he is less concerned with simplicity than with relevance. No matter how simple a message is, he said, "When we fail to couch our message in a framework that is personally relevant to the target audience, it has little prayer of ever penetrating to the point of changing behavior." He reiterated the need to understand who the target audience is and how to craft messages in a way that will be personally relevant to that audience. While public health professionals often want to communicate with everybody, which he called noble and virtuous, he said that using a single message to communicate with everybody is flawed from the outset.

7

Future Challenges and Solutions to Providing Healthy and Safe Foods to Aging Populations

The final session of the workshop began with a panel discussion aimed at highlighting the most important issues and future challenges to providing healthy and safe foods to aging populations. Moderators Susan Crockett of General Mills, Minneapolis, Minnesota, and Steven Gendel of the Food and Drug Administration's (FDA's) Center for Food Safety and Applied Nutrition (CFSAN), College Park, Maryland, introduced the four panelists: Pamela Starke-Reed, Deputy Director of the Division of Nutrition Research Coordination at the National Institutes of Health (NIH), Bethesda, Maryland; Johanna Dwyer, Senior Nutrition Scientist in the Office of Dietary Supplements (ODS) at NIH, Bethesda, Maryland, and Director of the Frances Stern Nutrition Center at Tufts University, Boston, Massachusetts; Jean Lloyd, National Nutritionist, Administration on Aging, U.S. Department of Health and Human Services (HHS), Washington, D.C.; and Dennis Sullivan, Director of Little Rock Geriatric Research, Education, and Clinical Center and Executive Vice Chairman of the Donald W. Reynolds Department of Geriatrics at the University of Arkansas for Medical Sciences, Little Rock, Arkansas.

Panelists considered a range of issues, from what one participant referred to as the "demographic imperative" (i.e., the large and fast-growing 65-and-over and 85-and-over populations) to the need for industry/government/academic collaborative efforts to improve nutrition communication to older consumers.

Issues included

- heterogeneity in the older population (with respect to age, race, income, functionality, family support, etc.) and the need to define what is meant when discussing "the older population";
- the need for more research on different subsets of the older population (e.g., on exposure levels and the risk of infection or illness from eating pathogen-contaminated foods) and the lack of sufficient population-level data for conducting that research;
- the likelihood that the scope of some food safety and nutrition-related problems in aging populations may be underestimated as a result of insufficient data;
- the need to more carefully consider the food safety and nutrition needs of the 85-and-over population, such as the diet quality of assisted living facility residents;
- the need for a stronger infrastructure and better nutrition services for older adults relying on home- or community-based care systems, particularly given that the "baby boom bubble" is moving across time and the 65 to 90 age group soon will represent a large proportion of the U.S. population;
- the need to reconsider the definition of an optimal diet for older adults, given changes in both physiology and eating habits;
- the need for more research on genetic variability and the potential importance of individualized nutrition (i.e., making dietary decisions based on genetic make-up);
- the need for more research on the value of probiotics in older adults' diets;
- the need for NIH and other government agencies to improve the way they communicate science to the public;
- the need to collaborate and involve the food industry in devising solutions to certain problems, such as communicating with older consumers and managing sodium intake in older adults' diets; and
- the need to consider how other countries are managing food safety and nutrition for older adults and whether the problems they encounter are similar.

An open dialogue with the audience followed the panel discussion, with the goal of discussing some of these and other challenges in detail and identifying possible solutions. In particular, workshop participants focused on

- the need to include nutrition education and communication in home- and community-based services for older adults;

- the importance of reducing sodium intake and the challenge of doing so with older adults;
- the need for more funding and stronger cross-sector collaborations (e.g., public-private) that have as one of their main goals addressing key unanswered questions about nutrition and food safety in aging populations;
- the need to balance apparently contradictory messages about food safety and nutrition (i.e., recommending that older adults eat or avoid certain foods as a way of maintaining long-term cardiovascular health while simultaneously warning about the risks of pathogen contamination in those same foods); and
- the challenge of communicating about food safety and nutrition in general with older adults.

Importantly, the goal of the panel discussion and open dialogue was not to reach consensus on any issue, including which issue(s) was considered most urgent. With some issues, there was a sense of general agreement among those voicing their opinions. With other issues, participants expressed varying opinions.

PANEL DISCUSSION

The Most Important and Urgent Issues

Gendel initiated the panel discussion with a deliberately unfocused question. He asked each panelist to elaborate on two or three issues that they considered the most important for follow up.

Starke-Reed mentioned several:

- She was struck by the heterogeneity of the aging population even with respect to age. For example, she observed that some presenters included all adults age 50 and over when discussing aging populations, whereas others considered only those age 65 and over. She stressed the importance of defining "aging population" in discussions because of this heterogeneity.
- She commented on some of the interesting research being conducted on probiotics and prebiotics and mentioned that NIH has a Roadmap Initiative focused on microorganisms. Her division at NIH has a working group devoted to researching the nutritive role of probiotics and prebiotics. She explained that there are 10,000 times as many bacterial cells as human cells in the human body and that

this is clearly an area of science that deserves the growing interest it is receiving.

- She commented on the lack of discussion around genetics and the importance of understanding whether individual genetic variation makes a difference in terms of optimizing nutrition for older adults. As with probiotics and prebiotics, research on nutrigenomics is also expanding not just at NIH but also at institutions worldwide.
- Finally, she stated that NIH is a research institution and does not do a very good job with "messaging." She said that NIH needs "a lot of help in that area." They need to know where they can send messages so that those messages can be translated and communicated to the appropriate population(s).

Dwyer commented on several points:

- She agreed with Starke-Reed that NIH must do a better job of communicating not just to the public but also to health care providers. For example, based on her work at the ODS, it is very important that information on the quality, safety, and efficacy of dietary supplements be effectively communicated to health care providers. While some supplements may be important or necessary for some older adults, others could be harmful. She encouraged workshop participants to visit the ODS website, remarking that it "is a very good piece of communication," but she said there is room for improvement.
- Like Starke-Reed, she was struck by some of the information on the demographics of aging populations. She said that she was particularly concerned with the 85-and-over population. She has been examining assisted living facilities for the past several years, and her research results have not been reassuring with respect to food safety. Food safety regulations vary from state to state, and nutrition regulations are practically nonexistent. The situation is very similar to what child daycare was like before it was regulated. She emphasized that this very important issue will need to be addressed soon, especially as the 85-and-over population becomes an increasingly large component of the aging population. Many people develop functional impairments when they reach the 85-and-over age group and are unable to live independently.
- Finally, she wondered when the United States is "going to wake up to the fact that we need a better system and a better infrastructure than we now have" for providing support to older community-dwelling adults who need assistance. She made this observation based on

her own personal situation with a 62-year old cousin who lives by herself and is suffering from multiple disabilities. She remarked that the issue is much broader than providing healthy and safe foods to aging populations.

Lloyd commented on a couple of issues:

- She agreed with the previous two panelists' comments about the heterogeneity of the aging population. Not only are there different age cohorts within "the aging population" but also different groups with varying needs (e.g., different incomes, varying amounts of family support).
- She expressed pleasure with the number of times that caregivers had been mentioned throughout the course of the workshop, given that the majority of elder care in the United States is provided by family caregivers. She noted that only 17 percent of the 85-and-older population is living in any kind of assisted care or other facility and that most of the "oldest old" remain community dwellers. Yet, while caregivers were mentioned at various times throughout the workshop, there was no discussion about how they should be providing the care. For example, most home- and community-based care systems do not have nutrition education components as Dwyer also mentioned. Like regulation of assisted living facilities, regulation of home- and community-based care is very fragmented, with different states imposing different sets of regulations. While some of the state-funded programs do have nutrition components, others do not. A major challenge is making all of this complex information about nutrition available to these caregivers in a way that enables the caretakers to make the best decisions. Meeting this challenge will be difficult given the lack of funding for home- and community-based care services and the long list of things that need to be done with that funding. Also, most home- and community-based care service programs are social service systems with limited awareness or understanding of nutrition and food safety.

Sullivan offered what he described as a "clinician perspective" on several key issues.

- He observed that not only are most older adults probably unaware of many food safety risks, but many health professionals do not fully comprehend the risks. There are many unanswered questions about individual variability, with respect to genetics as well as other factors. For example, many older patients have comorbid conditions or are taking medications that have profound physiological effects and can increase the risk of foodborne illness (e.g., people with age-related or drug-induced acid suppression are much more likely to have lower bowel infections; people on antibiotics are more susceptible to *Salmonella* and various other infections). He argued that in certain situations, there may be no cause for alarm and no reason to initiate a food recall on a national level, "we may be dramatically underestimating the significance of the problem on an individual basis, particularly when we are dealing with some of these very old patients." In other words, older patients may be at an even greater risk than the evidence suggests for the population at large. Complicating the problem is the fact that many older adults are unlikely to present with classic foodborne illness symptoms; in fact, they are more likely to present with confusion or other atypical symptoms. Also, older adults tend not to complain and do not like to discuss incontinence, diarrhea, and other similar problems with their physicians. Sullivan said that he personally would be paying more attention to food habits when dealing with older patients in the future.

- He commented on the fact that many older adults tend to be grazers and do not eat regular meals. This is particularly true of older women who live alone. Also, older adults tend to have fewer energy needs and therefore eat less. He said that for these and other reasons, as several previous speakers had alluded, "We have to rethink our ideas of what represents an optimal diet." For example, there are many unanswered questions about the role of supplements, such as how supplements should be manufactured (e.g., how they should be formulated), under what circumstances they are needed, and when they could be harmful. He stated that considerable evidence suggests that polymeric formulas may not be helpful in certain situations.
- He said that he was fascinated but also frightened by some of the demographic numbers presented during the workshop and the way the "baby boom bubble" is moving across time. Soon, the 65 to 90-year-old age group will represent a very large proportion of the U.S. population. That raises the question, "Who is going to be supporting them, particularly if they live to be 100, as a lot of people say they will?" The current U.S. infrastructure is predicated on the assumption that there will always be more workers than there are retired people, but what will happen when all the baby boomers retire? He also wondered about the social implications of the growing gap in life expectancy between females and males.

After the panelists reflected on what they thought were some of the important or interesting issues, the moderators voiced their opinions. Gendel observed that several speakers, as well as all four panelists, commented on the need to realize the tremendous heterogeneity of the "aging population" and the importance of differentiating among different subsets of older adults in order to better understand food safety risks. However, in reality this is difficult because of the lack of relevant data. He said, "We do in this country, by and large, a really bad job of monitoring health conditions and generating the kind of [population-level] information that would allow us to do that kind of impact analysis." It is very difficult to gather enough information on pathogen susceptibility such that it can be broken down and the relative susceptibilities of different subsets of older adults identified (e.g., susceptibilities of people 60 to 65 years old vs. people 85 and older). His point was that there is just not enough statistical information generated to allow for that kind of differentiation.

Crockett observed that the working model of the Food Forum is to bring academic, food industry, regulatory, and consumer representatives together to discuss common problems and identify potential solutions. This same model needs to be continued. She said, "I see enormous opportunity for the food industry to be part of the solution, but it won't happen unless we work very closely together." As just one example of how the food industry could contribute, she described a new community, Mill City Commons, forming in Minneapolis, Minnesota, where 50 to 55 year old empty nesters are moving into apartments downtown, close to the river, and are making provisions/plans to support themselves when they grow older and are in need of assistance. General Mills sees itself as a potential provider of foods for this type of "creative solution."

Lloyd remarked that Mill City Commons is an example of a naturally occurring retirement community (NORC). She stated that there is a large body of literature and many websites with information on NORCs, and in fact the Administration on Aging funds grants to support this type of livable community (not just for older adults but for other populations as well). She noted similar communities forming in Washington, DC and Boston. Crockett said that she was pleased to hear that Mill City Commons was part of a broader movement.

Questions Needing Answers

Crockett then asked the panelists if they had any remaining questions that they wish could be answered or would like to see answered through future research.

Starke-Reed stated that her main question is, "What is the optimal nutrition and diet for the older population?" Although there is some information available, she said, "We are really far from being able to define that right now."

Dwyer expressed concern in asking, "Where is the home and community-based older adult care system we keep hearing about?" She said that she did not want to downgrade current efforts, but the system at large is at the same place the United States was in the early years of the Roosevelt Administration with respect to children's services. She emphasized the need to develop the home- and community-based older adult care system so that it becomes more "coherent." She said that while the program in Boston's Beacon Hill is wonderful, there is no easily accessible comparable program in the Boston neighborhood where she lives. Lack of a coherent infrastructure poses a tremendous challenge for family members and others who are suddenly faced with the need to care for a parent or other older adult. Without that infrastructure, how are food safety and nutrition messages going to reach the large proportion of older adults still living in their homes?

Lloyd agreed that there is no infrastructure in place at the federal level and that the fragmented, multi-funded, state-by-state system that does exist creates terrific geographic as well as economic challenges. What can be done to improve the situation? For example, she administers an Alaskan program that delivers home meals by dogsled, which is difficult when the service provider is in one location and the client is 90 miles away. That is a "very real challenge," she said. It is an example of what she referred to as a "whole system problem."

As an example of a more specific problem, Lloyd raised the issue of sodium level in foods. She questioned what would happen if the sodium level in foods was reduced and older adults with a reduced sense of saltiness ended up adding way too much salt. She asked, "How do we help people who may salt their food and never know, like a younger person knows, that it is too salty?"

Sullivan said that he agreed with Gendel's earlier point about the need for more data on aging populations, particularly among adults age 80 and over, so that appropriate risk management can be conducted. Most disabilities and some of the least manageable health problems occur in people age 80 and over, and therefore it would be very helpful to have a better understanding of this population. He said, "We need more data and more systems for obtaining that data."

Both moderators voiced their opinions. Gendel observed that everything discussed during this workshop was focused on the situation in the United States, even though all of the various components and ingredients of foods come from all over the world and foods are moved in and out of countries in a much more integrated fashion than in the past. He emphasized the need to consider how foods are produced in other countries and what the safety issues are elsewhere, because those factors can impact domestic food safety and nutrition. He also questioned how other countries would define "the aging population" and whether they would segment their aging population into multiple susceptible subpopulations (e.g., 50-and-over vs. 65-and-over vs. 85-and-over) in the same way that U.S. experts would. He asked, "Are the assumptions that we are making here going to hold true in other countries?"

Finally, Crockett responded to Lloyd's observations about sodium. She said that General Mills and other companies are working hard to reduce sodium levels in foods and that sodium reduction efforts represent an area where industry, scientists, and regulators need to work together. Efforts at General Mills are predicated on the assumption that the best way to reduce sodium is in relatively slow, small steps done in a "stealth way." Announcing that sodium is being reduced sets up consumers for expectations that may not be true. She emphasized the importance of teaching consumers to "like and accept a lower sodium food" by making slow changes over time.

Crockett also commented on the "us against them" type of attitude that is so pervasive throughout the food industry, although she observed that it was not evident during this workshop. As an example, she pointed to the way that some scientists and communicators make statements such as, "Avoid processed foods." General statements like that, with undefined terms, create confusion not just among consumers but also health professionals. Messages need to be more precise since the term processed foods has different meanings to different people. The need for more precise communication around nutrition is another example of where cooperative efforts among industry, scientists, and others could be constructive.

Dwyer agreed that nobody has really defined "processed food" very well and that there are different types of processing with different nutritional and safety implications.

OPEN DISCUSSION[1]

Nutrition Services in Home- and Community-Based Services for Older Adults

Wellman said that she was delighted to hear the panelists comment on the emergence, albeit slow, of home- and community-based services for older adults. However, as she emphasized in her presentation, nutrition services (e.g., meals, counseling, and education) are often overlooked, taken for granted, or underfunded. She echoed other suggestions that the

[1] In this section, workshop speakers and panelists are identified by name. Other workshop participants (i.e., members of the audience) are not identified by name.

Institute of Medicine (IOM) Food and Nutrition Board establish a committee to examine the role of nutrition in home- and community-based elder services. Good nutrition services should be universally accessible to older adults, particularly if efforts are going to be directed toward keeping older adults in the community and out of nursing homes.

An audience member commented on the opportunity to incorporate nutrition services into NORCs now, while they are still emerging, rather than waiting until all of these naturally occurring retirement communities have been built and then trying to work nutrition services into them later. This remark prompted Lloyd to suggest that state dietetic associations learn more about how decisions are made regarding the nutrition aspects of state-provided home- and community-based older adult care services and become more involved in that process.

The Challenge of Reducing Sodium Intake

Pelchat remarked that she appreciated the panelists' comments about sodium and stated that familiarity plays a large role in how much salt people like in their food. People that become familiar with low sodium will start preferring low sodium. However, it is very easy to "slip" and revert to a preference for a high level of sodium. While it may take a month to become accustomed to low sodium, it takes only a few days of eating a high sodium diet to start preferring that high level again.

Pelchat also commented on the gate-keeping function she had mentioned in her presentation. While it becomes reduced in the oldest old, with people who have lost some of their gate-keeping function less able to detect spoilage or excessive salt, there is also an upside: the "oldest old" typically do not notice disagreeable characteristics of salt substitutes and therefore tend to find them okay. For example, potassium chloride, a popular salt substitute, has several negative sensory properties detectable by younger adults (e.g., a metallic or bitter taste). People who have lost some gate-keeping function do not notice those properties. The same is true of dietary supplements, with many younger adults complaining that dietary supplements taste like chemicals or vitamins but many older adults thinking that they are "just delicious."

An audience member remarked on the important technological challenges of reducing sodium in many foods. He said, "Very often it is easy for us to say, 'take the salt out,' without recognizing the technological and scientific challenges." He agreed with Crockett that a "true partnership" between industry and NIH with the goal of developing innovative ways to remove salt would serve the older population well.

This last comment prompted Dwyer to suggest that perhaps it is time for the IOM Food and Nutrition Board to consider an updated report on designing foods for the aging population, with a focus on safety as well as nutrition. She mentioned a 1989 IOM report that focused on designing foods for meeting the dietary guidelines. An audience member agreed, commenting on the need to include in any updated report all of the new technologies being applied to food design (e.g., nanotechnology).

More Data, Funding, and Cross-Sector Collaborations

Meydani stated that there are many unanswered questions about what constitutes optimal nutrition for older adults, how to communicate about nutrition with older adults, and how food products for older adults should be designed. However, research in any of these areas cannot be conducted without funding. She asked the panelists what efforts were being made to increase funding for this type of research and whether public-private partnerships would be helpful in providing some answers.

Starke-Reed replied that this is definitely an area of focus for the National Institute of Aging (NIA), although she did not know any details about the actual level of funding or whether plans were in place to increase funding. She said, "But it certainly is in their mission . . . and they do a fair amount of funding in that." Nutrition is a component of many of the other Institutes, besides NIA. However, she doubted that anyone at the Institutes would agree that funding for nutrition research is at the level it should be.

Starke-Reed also mentioned that while there are opportunities and avenues for NIH to collaborate with industry, it would be "really helpful for government" if industry would make the necessary information (which is otherwise proprietary) available so that it can be used to guide policy decision-making. She pointed to Wellman's use of proprietary data in her presentation as an example of how helpful those data can be.

Crockett remarked that at a previous Food Forum workshop on sodium reduction, several suggestions were made about possible ways that consumer behavior data could be shared with the U.S. Department of Agriculture (USDA) for nutrition monitoring. That discussion is ongoing and serves as just one example of an effort to initiate industry-government collaboration. She agreed that Wellman's use of General Mills' data is another.

While on the topic of data-sharing, Gendel remarked that the food industry generates a lot of data in areas such as quality assurance/quality control and sanitation that would be very useful for risk assessment and for understanding what exposure is occurring and the consequences of that exposure. However, it is very difficult to obtain those data. He mentioned several efforts being directed toward developing a way to share those data, but the problem has yet to be solved. He also mentioned the importance of negative test results. He says that he often hears industry representatives say that they have conducted thousands of tests a year and that "they all come up negative." From a risk assessment perspective, knowing that zero tests have come up negative is just as important as knowing that one test has come up positive. He said, "I wish there was a better way of getting some of those data."

In response to Crockett's earlier comments about the potentially very beneficial role that industry could play in addressing some challenges, Dwyer remarked that the food and perhaps equipment industries could help with communication around microwave wattage as earlier mentioned by Hallman (see Chapter 6). Given the increasing variety of microwaveable foods and the convenience and ease of using a microwave oven to heat food, the potential arises for inadequately cooked food, which has possible food safety implications. Many microwaveable food packages feature cooking instructions that vary depending on the wattage of the microwave used to heat the product. However, most people, not just older adults, do not know where wattage is indicated on their microwaves. "Yet," she said, "it is a simple food safety thing that could really perhaps make a difference with a lot of people." An audience member mentioned that the food industry, microwave manufacturers, and retailers are currently working on this issue and that wattage will be placed on the front of microwaves in the future.

Another audience member remarked on the "little rules" that exist around collaborating with industry. She said, "The minute you do that, then everybody starts saying you have lost your credibility." Another audience member commented on how industry is "very willing and open" to public-private partnerships but that a major challenge is the notion that industry has no credibility. He said that much of this attitude is historic and that it is time to move forward and create a new "framework" for partnership.

The Challenge of Communicating About Food Safety and Nutrition with Older Adults

An audience member expressed concern that most regulatory communication is directed to the general public and does not target specific subpopulations, like older adults. He asked how nutrition information that is of particular relevance to older adults should be communicated. Starke-Reed mentioned a past collaborative effort between NIA and the Grocery Manufacturers Association (GMA) that was aimed at older adult consumers, whereby NIA provided the science and GMA communicated the information in a consumer-friendly way. The program provided older consumers with information about foods that they should consider; changed the way products were located on shelves so that somebody did not have to reach up and grab a five-pound bag of sugar, worried that it might fall; etc. She cited it as an example of how nutrition science can be communicated directly to a specific population without going through any regulatory avenues.

Balancing Conflicting Messages About Food Safety vs. Nutrition

An audience member commented on how nutrition experts usually advise consumers to eat more fruits and vegetables, as a way to reduce their risk of chronic disease, while food safety experts express concern about foodborne disease originating from consumption of those very same foods (e.g., *E. coli* O157:H7 in spinach, *Salmonella* in tomatoes). She asked the panelists how the nutrition and food safety communities, which traditionally have not worked together, can work together to craft a message about the need to eat nutritiously while also keeping safety in mind.

Starke-Reed commented on the combined efforts of HHS and USDA in issuing the *Dietary Guidelines for Americans* and that those guidelines contain both food safety and nutrition information. Dwyer added that while considerable work was done in order to include the food safety guidelines in the 2000 *Dietary Guidelines for Americans*, the issue has "sort of gone underground" since then and that "it is time for that to come out again." Starke-Reed mentioned that the forthcoming *Dietary Guidelines'* subcommittee on food safety is "deliberating right now" and "would be very welcome" to comments. Lloyd mentioned that when the 2005 *Dietary Guidelines for Americans* were issued, a brochure designed specifically for older adults was also issued, with larger font sizes, artwork, and an emphasis on safety. The new guidelines should do the same.

An audience member remarked on need to "re-energize" the food safety program of the American Dietetic Association (ADA) and to do so with a focus on the older population.

Another audience member agreed that balancing messages about food safety and nutrition is very important. He said he is very concerned when he hears messages about the risks of eating fruits and vegetables given that the majority of older adults are going to die from chronic diseases, not foodborne illnesses. Today, not a single state "meets the basic guidelines for fruits and vegetables."

References

Bailey, R. L., J. H. Ledikwe, H. Smiciklas-Wright, D. C. Mitchell, and G. L. Jensen. 2004. Persistent oral health problems associated with co-morbidity and impaired diet quality in older adults. *Journal of the American Dietetic Association* 104(8):1273-1276.

Beck, M., P. C. Kolbeck, L. H. Rohr, Q. Shi, V. C. Morris, and O. A. Levander. 1994. Benign human enterovirus becomes virulent in selenium-deficient mice. *Journal of Medical Virology* 43(2):166-170.

Belisle, S. E., L. S. Leka, J. Delgado-Lista, P. F. Jacques, J. M. Ordovas, and S. N. Meydani. 2009. Polymorphisms at cytokine genes may determine the effect of vitamin E on cytokine production in the elderly. *Journal of Nutrition* 139(10):1855-1860.

Bernhard, D., and G. Laufer. 2008. The aging cardiomyocyte: A mini-review. *Gerontology* 54(1):24-31.

Bernstein, M. E., K. L. Tucker, N. D. Ryan, E. F. O'Neill, K. M. Clements, M. E. Nelson, W. J. Evans, and M. A. F. Singh. 2002. Higher dietary variety is associated with better nutritional status in frail elderly people. *Journal of the American Dietetic Association* 102(8):1096-1104.

Blaser, M. J. and R. A. Feldman. 1981. *Salmonella* bacteremia: Reports to the Centers for Disease Control, 1968-1979. *Journal of Infectious Diseases* 143(5):743-746.

Blom, H., E. Nerbrink, R. Dainty, T. Hagtvedt, E. Borch, H. Nissen, and T. Nesbakkehn. 1997. Addition of 2.5 percent lactate and 0.25 percent acetate controls growth of *Listeria monocytogenes* in vacuum-packed, sensory-acceptable servelat sausage and cooked ham stored at 4 degrees C. *International Journal of Food Microbiology* 38(1):71-76.

Breece, C. R., R. L. Ingram, and W. E. Sonntag. 1991. Influence of age and long-term dietary restriction on plasma insulin-like growth factor-1 (IGF-1), IGF-1 gene expression, and IGF-1 binding proteins. *Journal of Gerontology* 46(5):B180-B187.

Buell, J. S., T. M. Scott, B. Dawson-Hughes, G. E. Dallal, I. H. Rosenberg, M. F. Foldstein, and K. L. Tucker. 2009. Vitamin D is associated with cognitive function in elders receiving home health services. *Journal of Gerontology Series A: Biological Sciences and Medical Sciences* 64(8):888-895.

Cain, W. S. and J. C. Stevens. 1989. Uniformity of olfactory loss in aging. *Annals of the New York Academy of Sciences* 561:29-38.

Calle, E. E., M. J. Thun, J. M. Petrelli, C. Rodriguez, and C. W. Heath. 1999. Body-mass index and mortality in a prospective cohort of U.S. adults. *New England Journal of Medicine* 341(15):1097-1105.

Cavaliere, C., P. Rea, M. E. Lynch, and M. Blumenthal. 2009. Herbal supplement sales experience slight increase in 2008. *HerbalGram* 82:58-61.

CDC (Centers for Disease Control and Prevention). 2010. Vital signs: State-specific obesity prevalence among adults—United States, 2009. *Morbidity and Mortality Weekly Report* 59:1-5.

Chan, J. M., M. J. Stampfer, E. Giovannucci, P. H. Gann, J. Ma, P. Wilkinson, C. H. Hennekens, and M. Pollak. 1998. Plasma insulin-like growth factor-1 and prostate cancer risk: A prospective study. *Science* 279:563-566.

Clark, C. G., J. Farber, F. Pagotto, N. Ciampa, K. Dore, C. Nadon, K. Bernard, and L. K. Ng. 2010. Surveillance for *Listeria monocytogenes* and listeriosis, 1995-2004. *Epidemiology and Infection* 138(4):559-572.

Colman, R. J., R. M. Anderson, S. C. Johnson, E. K. Kastman, K. J. Kosmatka, T. M. Beasley, D. B. Allison, C. Cruzen, H. A. Simmons, J. W. Kemnitz, and R. Weindruch. 2009. Caloric restriction delays disease onset and mortality in rhesus monkeys. *Science* 325(5937):201-204.

CSPI (Center for Science in the Public Interest). 2008. *Dirty Dining*. Washington, DC: CSPI.

Cuite, C. L., S. C. Condry, M. L. Nucci, and W. K. Hallman. 2007. Public response to the contaminated spinach recall of 2006. Publication number RR-0107-013. New Brunswick, NJ: Rutgers, the State University of New Jersey, Food Policy Institute.

Cuite, C. L., S. D. Schefske, E. M. Randolph, N. H. Hooker, M. L. Nucci, and W. K. Hallman. 2008. Public response to the *Salmonella* Saintpaul outbreak of 2008. Publication number RR-1208-017. New Brunswick, NJ: Rutgers, the State University of New Jersey, Food Policy Institute.

Cummings, S. R. 2007. The biology of aging. *Journal of Musculoskeletal and Neuronal Interactions* 7(4):340-341.

D'Archivio, M., C. Filesi, R. Varì, B. Scazzocchio, and R. Masella. 2010. Bioavailability of the pholyphenols: Status and controversies. *International Journal of Molecular Sciences* 11(4):1321-1342.

Daly, K. T., A. C. Tracy, M. Malik, T. Wang, S. Francke-Carroll, and B. A. Magnuson. 2007. Enhanced estrogenic responses and sensitivity to azoxymethane following dietary soy isoflavone supplementation in older female rats. *Food and Chemical Toxicology* 45(4):628-637.

Dundas, S., W. T. Todd, A. L. Stewart, P. S. Murdoch, A. K. Chaudhuri, and S. J. Hutchinson. 2001. The central Scotland *Escherichia coli* O157:H7 outbreak: Risk factors for the hemolytic uremic syndrome and death among hospitalized patients. *Clinical Infectious Diseases* 33(7):923-931.

Edgar, B., D. Bailey, R. Bergstrand, G. Johnsson, and C. G. Regårdh. 1992. Acute effects of drinking grapefruit juice on the pharmacokinetics and dynamics of felodipine—and its potential clinical relevance. *European Journal of Clinical Pharmacology* 42(3):313-317.

FDA/HHS (U.S. Food and Drug Administration/Department of Health and Human Services). 2007. Food labeling: Revision of reference values and mandatory nutrients. Advance notice of proposed rulemaking. *Federal Register* 72(212):62149-62174.

Fontana, L., T. E. Meyer, S. Klein, and J. O. Holloszy. 2004. Long-term calorie restriction is highly effective in reducing the risk for atherosclerosis in humans. *Proceedings of the National Academy of Sciences* 101(17):6659-6663.

Fontana, L., E. P. Weiss, D. T. Villareal, S. Klein, and J. O. Holloszy. 2008. Long-term effects of calorie or protein restriction on serum IGF-1 and IGFBP-3 concentration in humans. *Aging Cell* 7(5):681-687.

Fontana, L., S. Klein, and J. O. Holloszy. 2009. Effects of long-term calorie restriction and endurance exercise on glucose intolerance, insulin action, and adipokine production. *Age* 32(1):97-108.

Gay, R. T., S. Belisle, M. A. Beck, and S. N. Meydani. 2006. An aged host promotes the evolution of avirulent coxsackievirus into a virulent strain. *Proceedings of the National Academy of Sciences* 103(37):13825-13830.

Ginsberg, G., D. Hattis, A. Russ, and B. Sonawane. 2005. Pharmacokinetic and pharmacodynamic factors that can affect sensitivity to neurotoxic sequelae in elderly individuals. *Environmental Health Perspectives* 113(9):1243-1249.

Greenblatt, D. J. 2010. Update on drug interactions with grapefruit juice. *Pharmacy Times* [Continuing Education] 76:95-104.

Hallman, W. K., C. L. Cuite, and N. H. Hooker. 2009. Consumer responses to food recalls: 2008 national survey report. Publication number RR-0109-018. New Brunswick, NJ: Rutgers, the State University of New Jersey, Food Policy Institute.

Hankinson, S. E., W. C. Willett, G. A. Colditz, D. J. Hunter, D. S. Michaud, B. Deroo, B. Rosner, F. E. Speizer, and M. Pollak. 1998. Circulating concentrations of insulin-like growth factor-1 and risk of breast cancer. *Lancet* 351(9113):1393-1396.

Hannan, M. T., K. L. Tucker, B. Dawson-Hughes, L. A. Cupples, D. T. Felson, and D. P. Kiel. 2000. Effect of dietary protein on bone loss in elderly men and women: the Framingham osteoporosis study. *Journal of Bone and Mineral Research* 15(12):2504-2512.

Hayek, M. G., S. N. Meydani, M. Meydani, and J. B. Blumberg. 1994. Age differences in eicosanoid production of mouse splenocytes: Effects on mitogen-induced T-cell proliferation. *Journal of Gerontology* 49(5):B197-207.

Healton, E. B., D. G. Savage, J. C. M. Brust, T. J. Garrett, and J. Lindenbaum. 1991. Neurologic aspects of cobalamin deficiency. *Medicine* 70(4):229-245.

Hickson, M. 2006. Malnutrition and ageing. *Postgraduate Medical Journal* 82(963):2-8.

Holloszy, J. O. 1997. Mortality rate and longevity of food-restricted exercising male rats: A reevaluation. *Journal of Applied Physiology* 82(2):399-403.

Hopkins, M. J. and C. G. Macfarlane. 2002. Changes in predominant bacterial populations in human feces with age and with Clostridium difficile infection. *Journal of Medical Microbiology* 51(5):448-454.

Houston, D. K., B. J. Nicklas, J. Ding, T. B. Harris, F. A. Tylavsky, A. B. Newman, J. S. Lee, N. R. Sahyoun, M. Visser, and S. B. Kritchevsky. 2008. Dietary protein intake is associated with lean mass change in older, community-dwelling adults: The Health, Aging, and Body Composition (Health ABC) Study. *American Journal of Clinical Nutrition* 87(1):150-155.

Hu, F. B., W. C. Willett, T. Li, M. J. Stampfer, G. A. Colditz, and J. E. Manson. 2004. Adiposity as compared with physical activity in predicting mortality among women. *New England Journal of Medicine* 351(26):2694-2703.

IFIC (International Food Information Council). 2009. Food & Health Survey: Consumer Attitudes toward Food, Nutrition & Health. Washington, DC: International Food Information Council Foundation.

IOM (Institute of Medicine). 1994. *Nutrition and Food Sciences*. Washington, DC: National Academy Press.

IOM. 2005. *Dietary Reference Intakes for Energy, Carbohydrate, Fiber, Fat, Fatty Acids, Cholesterol, Protein, and Amino Acids (Macronutrients)*. Washington, DC: The National Academies Press.

IOM. 2006. *Dietary Reference Intakes: The essential guide to nutrient requirements.* Edited by J. J. Otten, J. P. Hellwig, and L. D. Meyers. Washington, DC: The National Academies Press.

Kamp, B. J., N. S. Wellman, and C. Russell. 2010. Position of the American Dietetic Association, American Society for Nutrition, and Society for Nutrition Education: Food and nutrition programs for community-residing older adults. *Journal of the American Dietetic Association* 110(3):463-472.

Kwan, L. L., O. I. Bermudez, and K. L. Tucker. 2002. Low vitamin B_{12} intake and status are more prevalent in Hispanic older adults of Caribbean origin than in neighborhood-matched non-Hispanic whites. *Journal of Nutrition* 132(7):2059-2064.

Kwon, Y., and B. A. Magnuson. 2007. Aging alters acute apoptotic response to azoxymethane in the colon of rats. *Experimental Gerontology* 42(12):1154-1161.

Kwon, Y., and B. A. Magnuson. 2009. Age-related differential responses to curcumin-induced apoptosis during the initiation of colon cancer in rats. *Food Chemical Toxicology* 47(2):377-385.

Kwon, Y., M. Malik, and B. A. Magnuson. 2004. Inhibition of colonic aberrant crypt foci by curcumin in rats is affected by age. *Nutrition and Cancer* 48(1):37-43.

Lianou, A., I. Geornaras, P. A. Kendall, J. A. Scanga, and J. N. Sofos. 2007. Behavior of *Listeria monocytogenes* at 7 degrees C in commercial turkey breast, with or without antimicrobials, after simulated contamination for manufacturing, retail and consumer settings. *Food Microbiology* 24(5):433-443.

Lichtenstein, A. H., H. Rasmussen, W. W. Yu, S. R. Epstein, and R. M. Russell. 2008. Modified MyPyramid for older adults. *Journal of Nutrition* 138(1):5-11.

Lilja, J. J., K. T. Kivisto, J. T. Backman, T. S. Lamberg, and P. J. Neuvonen. 1998. Grapefruit juice substantially increases plasma concentrations of buspirone. *Clinical Pharmacology and Therapeutics* 64(6):655-660.

Loya, A. M., A. Gonzalez-Stuart, and J. O. Rivera. 2009. Prevalence of polypharmacy, polyherbacy, nutritional supplement use and potential product interactions among older adults living on the United States-Mexico border: A descriptive, questionnaire-based study. *Drugs and Aging* 26(5):423-436.

McFarland, L. V. 2006. Meta-analysis of probiotics for the prevention of antibiotic associated diarrhea and the treatment of *Clostridium difficile* disease. *The American Journal of Gastroenterology* 101(4):812-822.

McFarland, L. V. 2010. Systematic review and meta-analysis of *Saccharromyces boulardii* in adult patients. *World Journal of Gastroenterology* 16(18):2202-2222.

Merete, C., L. M. Falcon, and K. L. Tucker. 2008. Vitamin B_6 is associated with depressive symptomatology in Massachusetts elders. *Journal of the American College of Nutrition* 27(3):421-427.

Meydani, S. N., J. D. Ribaya-Mercado, R. M. Russell, N. Sahyoun, F. D. Morrow, and S. N. Gershoff. 1990. The effect of vitamin B_6 on the immune response of healthy elderly. *Annals of the New York Academy of Sciences* 587:303-306.

Meydani, S. N., A. H. Lichtenstein, S. Cornwall, M. Meydani, B. R. Goldin, H. Rasmussen, C. A. Dinarello, and E. J. Schaefer. 1993. Immunologic effects of national cholesterol education panel step-2 diets with and without fish-derived N-3 fatty acid enrichment. *Journal of Clinical Investigation* 92(1):105-113.

Meydani, S. N., M. Meydani, J. B. Blumberg, L. S. Leka, G. Siber, R. Loszewski, C. Thompson, M. C. Pedrosa, R. D. Diamond, and B. D. Stollar. 1997. Vitamin E supplementation and in vivo immune response in healthy elderly subjects. A randomized controlled trial. *Journal of the American Medical Association* 277(17):1380-1386.

Meydani, S. N., L. S. Keka, B. C. Fine, G. E. Dallal, G. T. Keusch, M. F. Singh, and D. H. Hamer. 2004. Vitamin E and respiratory tract infections in elderly nursing home residents: A randomized controlled trial. *Journal of the American Medical Association* 292(7):828-836.

Meydani, S. N., J. B. Barnett, G. E. Dallal, B. C. Fine, P. F. Jacques, L. S. Leka, and D. H. Hamer. 2007. Serum zinc and pneumonia in nursing home elderly. *American Journal of Clinical Nutrition* 86(4):1167-1173.

Murphy, C., C. R. Schubert, K. J. Cruickshanks, B. E. Klein, R. Klein, and D. M. Nondahl. 2002. Prevalence of olfactory impairment in older adults. *Journal of the American Medical Association* 288(18):2307-2312.

Newby, P. K., D. Muller, J. Hallfrisch, N. Qiao, R. Andres, and K. L. Tucker. 2003. Dietary patterns and changes in body mass index and waist circumference in adults. *American Journal of Clinical Nutrition* 77(6):1417-1425.

Nucci, M. L., C. L. Cuite, and W. K. Hallman. 2009. When good food goes bad: Television network news and the spinach outbreak of 2006. *Science Communication* 31(2):238-265.

Ogden, C. L., M. D. Carroll, L. R. Curtin, M. A. McDowell, C. J. Tabak, and K. M. Flegal. 2006. Prevalence of overweight and obesity in the United States, 1999–2004. *The Journal of the American Medical Association* 295(13):1549-1555.

Pallast, E. G., E. G. Schouten, F. G. de Waart, H. C. Fonk, G. Doekes, B. M. von Blomberg, and F. J. Kok. 1999. Effect of 50- and 100-mg vitamin E supplements on cellular immune function in noninstitutionalized elderly persons. *American Journal of Clinical Nutrition* 69(6):1273-1281.

Pelchat, M. L. 2001. Is age-related olfactory loss uniform across odorants? In *Compendium of Olfactory Research*, edited by T. S. Lorig. Dubuque, Iowa: Kendall/Hunt Publishing Company. Pp 3-12.

Peterson, R. T., R. Nass, W. A. Boyd, J. H. Freedman, K. Dong, and T. Narahashi. 2008. Use of non-mammalian alternative models for neurotoxicological study. *Neurotoxicology* 29(3):546-555.

Rand, W. M., P. L. Pellett, and V. R. Young. 2003. Meta-analysis of nitrogen balance studies for estimating protein requirements in healthy adults. *American Journal of Clinical Nutrition* 77(1):109-127.

Ren, Z., R. Gay, A. Thomas, M. Pae, D. Wu, L. Logsdon, J. Mecsas, and S. N. Meydani. 2009. Effect of age on susceptibility to *Salmonella* Typhimurium infection in C57BL/6 mice. *Journal of Medical Microbiology* 58(Pt12):1559-1567.

Russell, R. M., H. Rasmussen, and A. H. Lichtenstein. 1999. Modified food guide pyramid for people over seventy years of age. *Journal of Nutrition* 129(3):751-753.

Saper, R. B., S. N. Kales, J. Paquin, M. J. Burns, D. M. Eisenberg, R. B. Davis, and R. S. Phillips. 2004. Heavy metal content of ayurvedic herbal medicine products. *Journal of the American Medical Association* 292(23):2868-2873.

Schiffman, S. 2009. Effects of aging on the human taste system. *Annals of the New York Academy of Sciences* 1170:725-729.

Schmelz, E. M., E. Levi, J. Du, H. Xu, and A. P. Majumdar. 2004. Age-related loss of EGF-receptor related protein (ERRP) in the aging colon is a potential risk factor for colon cancer. *Mechanisms of Ageing and Development* 125(12):917-922.

Shatenstein, B., H. Payette, S. Nadon, and K. Gray-Donald. 2003. An approach for evaluating lifelong intakes of functional foods in elderly people. *Journal of Nutrition* 133(7):2384-2391.

Shimokawa, I., Y. Higami, G. B. Hubbard, C. A. McMahan, E. J. Masoro, and B. P. Yu. 1993. Diet and the suitability of the male Fischer 344 rat as a model for aging research. *Journal of Gerontology* 48(1):B27-B32.

Shu, C. H., T. Hummel, P. L. Lee, C. H. Chiu, S. H. Lin, and B. C. Yuan. 2009. The proportion of self-rated olfactory dysfunction does not change across the life-span. *American Journal of Rhinology and Allergy* 23(4):413-416.

Sivapalasingam, S., R. M. Hoekstra, J. R. McQuiston, P. I. Fields, and R. V. Tauxe. 2004. *Salmonella* bacteriuria: an increasing entity in elderly women in the United States. *Epidemiology and Infection* 132(5):897-902.

Soliman, N., M. el-Batran, and A. el-Nofely. 1999. Oral health and nutritional status in Egyptian elderly. *Journal of Nutritional Science and Vitaminology* 45(5):533-541.

Sullivan, D. H., W. Martin, N. Flaxman, and J. E. Hagen. 1993. Oral health problems and involuntary weight loss in a population of frail elderly. *Journal of the American Geriatrics Society* 41(7):725-731.

Talegawkar, S. A., E. J. Johnson, T. Carithers, H. A. Taylor Jr., M. L. Bogle, and K. L. Tucker. 2007. Total alpha-tocopherol intakes are associated with serum alpha-tocopherol concentrations in African American adults. *Journal of Nutrition* 137(10):2297-2303.

Thaler, R. H. and C.S. Sunstein. 2004. *Nudge: Improving Decisions about Health, Wealth, and Happiness*. Penguin Books, USA.

Tucker, K. L., S. Rich, I. Rosenberg, P. Jacques, G. Dallal, P. W. Wilson, and J. Selhub. 2000. Plasma vitamin B-12 concentrations relate to intake source in the Framingham Offspring Study. *American Journal of Clinical Nutrition* 71(2):514-522.

Tucker, K. L., N. Qiao, T. Scott, I. Rosenberg, and A. Spiro, III. 2005. High homocysteine and low B vitamins predict cognitive decline in aging men: The Veterans Affairs Normative Aging Study. *American Journal of Clinical Nutrition* 82(3):627-635.

USDA (U.S. Department of Agriculture). 2009. Economic Information Bulletin No. (EIB-61), Food Spending Declined and Food Insecurity Increased for Middle-Income and Low-Income Households from 2000 to 2007, www.ers.usda.gov/Publications/EIB61 (accessed August 5, 2010).

Vugia, D., A. Cronquist, M. Cartter, M. Tobin-D'Angelo, D. Blythe, K. Smith, S. Lathrop, D. Morse, P. Cieslak, J. Dunn, K. G. Holt, O. L. Henao, R. M. Hoekstra, F. J. Angulo, P. M. Griffin, R. V. Tauxe, and K. K. Trivedi. 2009. Preliminary FoodNet data on the incidence of infection with pathogens transmitted commonly through food—10 states, 2008. *Morbidity and Mortality Weekly Report* 58(13):333-337.

Weimer, J. R. 1997. Many elderly at nutritional risk. *USDA Food Review* 20(1):42-48.

Weindruch, R. and R. S. Sohal. 1997. Seminars in medicine of the Beth Israel Deaconess Medical Center: Caloric intake and aging. *New England Journal of Medicine* 337(14):986-994.

Weindruch, R. and R. L. Walford. 1982. Dietary restriction in mice beginning at 1 year of age: Effect on life-span and spontaneous cancer incidence. *Science* 215(4538):1415-1418.

Weisskopf, M. G., N. Jain, H. Nie, D. Sparrow, P. Vokonas, J. Schwartz, and H. Hu. 2009. A prospective study of bone lead concentrations and death from all causes, cardiovascular diseases, and cancer in the Department of Veteran Affairs Normative Aging Study. *Circulation* 120(12):1056-1064.

Willett, W. C., W. H. Dietz, and G. A. Colditz. 1999. Guidelines for healthy weight. *New England Journal of Medicine* 341(6):427-434.

Woodmansey, E. J. 2007. Intestinal bacteria and ageing. *Journal of Applied Microbiology* 102(5):1178-1186.

Wu, D., S. N. Han, M. Meydani, and S. N. Meydani. 2006. Effect of concomitant consumption of fish oil and vitamin E on T cell-mediated function in the elderly: A randomized double-blind trial. *Journal of the American College of Nutrition* 25(4):300-306.

Wysocki, C. J. and A. N. Gilbert. 1989. National Geographic smell survey. Effects of age are heterogeneous. *Annals of the New York Academy of Sciences* 561:12-28.

Zhao, T., P. Zhao, and M. P. Doyle. 2009. Inactivation of *Salmonella* and *Escherichia coli* O157:H7 on lettuce and poultry skin by combination of levulinic acid and sodium dodecyl sulfate. *Journal of Food Protection* 72(5):928-936.

Zhu, Y, L. Gu, J. Yu, J. Yang, X. Zhai, C. Dong, H. Qian, Z. Tan, H. Pan, J. Liu, F. Zhu, and H. Wang. 2009. Analysis on the epidemiological characteristics of *Escherichia coli* O157: H7 infection in Zuzhou, Jiangsu, China, 1999. *Journal of Nanjing Medical University* 23(1):20-24.

A

Workshop Agenda

The National Academy of Sciences Building
Auditorium
2100 C Street NW
Washington, DC

October 29, 2009

8:00 am *Registration*

INTRODUCTION

8:30 **Welcome from the Food Forum**
Michael Doyle, Food Forum Chair, University of Georgia

8:40 **Opening Remarks—Overview of the Challenges to Ensuring Safe and Nutritious Foods for Aging Populations**
Stephen Sundlof, Food and Drug Administration

SESSION 1: SIZE AND DEMOGRAPHICS OF AGING POPULATIONS

Moderator: *Pamela Starke-Reed, National Institutes of Health*

9:00 **Our Aging Population**
Kevin Kinsella, National Institute on Aging

9:30 **Food Preparation and Consumption Habits of Community–Dwelling Populations**
Nancy Wellman, Tufts University

10:00 **Questions and Discussion**

10:30 ***Break***

SESSION 2: CHANGES IN PHYSIOLOGY WITH AGE

Moderator: *Gordon Jensen, Pennsylvania State University*

10:45 **Immune Status of Aging Populations and Methods of Modulating Susceptibility**
Simin Meydani, Jean Mayer USDA–Human Nutrition Research Center on Aging at Tufts University

11:05 **Gastrointestinal System Changes with Age**
Gordon Jensen, Pennsylvania State University

11:25 **Sensory Perception Changes with Age**
Marcia Pelchat, Monell Chemical Senses Center

11:45 **Questions and Discussion**

12:15 pm ***Lunch***

SESSION 3: FOOD SAFETY CONCERNS FOR AGING POPULATIONS

Moderator: *Kerry Dearfield, U.S. Department of Agriculture*

1:00 **Pathogens of Concern**
Steven Gendel, Food and Drug Administration

1:20 **Contaminants of Concern**
Bernadene Magnuson, Cantox Health Sciences International

1:40 **Processing and Formulation Advances to Decrease Food Safety Risks**
Michael Doyle, University of Georgia

2:00 **Packaging and Storage Challenges and Solutions to Decreasing Safety Risks**
Aaron Brody, Packaging/Brody, Inc.

2:20 **Panel Discussion on Implications for Regulators, Educators, and the Food Industry**
All Speakers and David J. Greenblatt, Tufts University

3:10 ***Break***

SESSION 4: NUTRITION CONCERNS FOR AGING POPULATIONS

Moderator: *Johanna Dwyer, National Institutes of Health and Tufts University*

3:30 **Diet Quality Issues for Aging Populations**
Katherine Tucker, Jean Mayer USDA-Human Nutrition Research Center on Aging at Tufts University

3:50 **Functional Foods and Aging Populations**
Stephen Barnes, University of Alabama at Birmingham

4:10 **Nutritional Modulation of Aging and Age-Associated Diseases by Caloric Restriction**
Luigi Fontana, Washington University and Italian National Institute of Health

4:30 **Formulating for Aging Boomer Consumers**
Jim Kirkwood, General Mills

4:50 **Panel Discussion on Implications for Regulators, Educators, and the Food Industry**
All Speakers

5:30 ***Adjourn***

October 30, 2009

SESSION 5: COMMUNICATING WITH AGING POPULATIONS

Moderator: *Edward Groth, Groth Consulting Services*

8:30 am **Consumer Desires, Needs, and Motivations**
Steven Bodhaine, The Futures Company

8:50 **Food Safety Messages—What do Consumers Hear?**
Caroline Smith DeWaal, Center for Science in the Public Interest

9:10 **Communicating with Older Consumers During Recalls**
William Hallman, Rutgers University

9:30 **Communicating Nutrition Messages to Older Persons**
Ronni Chernoff, Geriatric Research Education and Clinical Center, John L. McClellan Memorial Veterans Hospital in Little Rock, Arkansas

9:50 **Questions and Discussion**

10:30 ***Break***

SESSION 6: FUTURE CHALLENGES AND SOLUTIONS TO PROVIDING HEALTHY AND SAFE FOODS TO AGING POPULATIONS

11:00 **Panel Discussion**

Moderators:
Susan Crockett, General Mills
Steven Gendel, Food and Drug Administration

Panelists:
Pamela Starke-Reed, National Institutes of Health
Johanna Dwyer, National Institutes of Health and Tufts University
Jean Lloyd, Administration on Aging
Dennis Sullivan, University of Arkansas for Medical Sciences

11:45 **Open Discussion**

12:30 pm ***Adjourn***

B

Workshop Participants

Joseph Albright
EPA
Washington, DC

Sarah Alligood
IFIC
Washington, DC

Carlos Alvarez Antolinez
European Commission Delegation
Washington, DC

Amy Anderson
University of Maryland
College Park, MD

James Astwood
Martek Biosciences
Columbia, MD

Charles Baker
The Sugar Association, Inc.
Washington, DC

Brian Barrows
Naval Research Laboratory
Washington, DC

Susan Berkow
SEB Associates
Alexandria, VA

Odilia Bermudez
Tufts University School of Medicine
Boston, MA

Donna Blum-Kemelor
USDA/CNPP
Alexandria, VA

Caitlin Boon
IOM
Washington, DC

Susan Borra
Edlelman
Washington, DC

Adriene Bortz
Genesis HealthCare
Food and Nutrition Services

Mary Brandt
FDA/CFSAN
College Park, MD

Wendy Braund
DHHS/ODPHP
Rockville, MD

Helen Brown
AARP
Washington, DC

Francis Busta
University of Minnesota
St. Paul, MN

Kristina Butts
National Cattlemen's Beef Association
Washington, DC

Mark Byron
Supplemental Food Programs/SFMNP
Alexandria, VA

Laurenda Carter
FDA
Laurel, MD

Jasmine Chan
Virginia Tech

Velma Charles-Shannon
USDA
Washington, DC

Alex Chasick
Consumers Union

Hongda Chen
USDA/CSREES
Washington, DC

Rhoda Cohen
Mathematica Policy Research, Inc.
Princeton, NJ

Thomas Collins
FDA (Retired)
Chevy Chase, MD

Bernadine Cruz
Lewis Center, OH

Marjorie Davidson
FDA/CFSAN
College Park, MD

Eric Decker
University of Massachusetts, Amherst
Amherst, MA

Mark Denbaly
USDA/ERS
Beltville, MD

Manashi Dey
FDA
Laurel, MD

Bob Dole
DoD Veterinary Service Activity
Falls Church, VA

Michael Doyle
University of Georgia
Griffin, GA

Johanna Dwyer
NIH/ODS
Bethesda, MD

Eileen Dykes
USDA/FSIS
Washington, DC

Nancy Emenaker
NIH/NCI
Rockville, MD

Michelle Everett
USDA/FSIS
Beltsville, MD

Shelley Feist
Partnership for Food Safety Education
Washington, DC

Faye Feldstein
FDA
Severna Park, MD

William Fisher
IFT
Washington, DC

Sheila Fleischhacker
University of North Carolina
Chapel Hill, NC

Tony Flood
IFIC
Washington, DC

Janet Gamble
EPA
Washington, DC

Steven Gendel
FDA/CFSAN
College Park, MD

Shirley Gerrior
USDA

Lisa Goodson
American University
Bethesda, MD

Mary Gorski
The Pew Charitable Trusts
Washington, DC

Marcia Greenblum
Egg Nutrition Center
Park Ridge, IL

Edward Groth
Groth Consulting Services
Pelham, NY

Mary Hager
ADA
Washington, DC

Brenda Halbrook
USDA/FNS
Alexandria, VA

Darlene Hardie-Muncy
Cargill
Wayzata, MN

Virginia Hartmuller
NIH/NCI
Ellicott City, MD

Jabari Hawkins
USDA/FSIS
Beltsville, MD

Eric Hentges
ILSI North America
Washington, DC

John Hicks
USDA/FSIS/OPPD
Beltsville, MD

Answorth Honore
Harris Methodist Hospital
Fort Worth, TX

Kelly Horton
Connect Nutrition

Van Hubbard
NIH/DNRC
Bethesda, MD

Jing Hu
University of Maryland
College Park, MD

Jayasri Janakiram
Children's Hospital
Washington, DC

Wendy Johnson-Askew
NIH
Bethesda, MD

Satya Jonnalagadda
General Mills Inc.
Golden Valley, MN

WenYen Juan
ONLDS/NPS
College Park, MD

Setsuko Kamotani
IFIC
Washington, DC

Mark Kantor
University of Maryland
College Park, MD

Joanne Karimbakas
American Institutes for Research
Silver Spring, MD

Teresa Keenan
AARP
Washington, DC

Kathleen Koehler
DHHS
Washington, DC

Connye Kuratko
Martek Biosciences
Columbia, MD

Alan Kurz
Consultant
Philadelphia, PA

Heejeong Latimer
USDA/FSIS
Washington, DC

Marie Latulippe
ILSI North America
Washington, DC

Christina Lengyel
University of Manitoba
Winnipeg, Manitoba

Jada Lewis
FDA/CFSAN
College Park, MD

Jeffrey Lewis
Prince George's County
Largo, MD

Jean Lloyd
USDA
Washington, DC

Andrew Maccabe
CDC
Washington, DC

Somdat Mahabir
NIH/NCI
Bethesda, MD

Amal Mahfouz
EPA
Washington, DC

Marilee Marchelya
University of Illinois
Winfield, IL

Ben Mathews
European Commission Delegation
Washington, DC

Melanie Mayor
FDA/CFSAN
College Park, MD

Erica McCoy
USDA
Washington, DC

Crystal McDade-Ngutter
NIH
Bethesda, MD

Meisha McDaniel
Congressional Hunger Center
Washington, DC

Holly McPeak
HHS/ODPHP
Rockville, MD

Mary McPhail Gray
USDA-REE
Washington, DC

Bernard Merkel
European Commission Delegation
Washington, DC

Stephanie Mickelson
USDA/FNS
Alexandria, VA

Marianne Miliotis
FDA/CFSAN
College Park, MD

John Milner
NIH/NCI
Rockville, MD

Suruchi Mishra
University of Maryland
College Park, MD

Karol Moen
Montgomery County Government

Patricia Montgomery
Campbell Soup Company
Camden, NJ

Sylvia Montgomery
USDA/CSREES
Washington, DC

Melissa Musiker
GMA
Washington, DC

Esther Myers
ADA
Chicago, IL

Keeve Nachman
Johns Hopkins University
Baltimore, MD

Joyce Njoroge
FDA
Laurel, MD

Sarah Ohlhorst
Institute of Food Technologists
Washington, DC

Erik Olson
The Pew Charitable Trusts
Washington, DC

Maria Oria
IOM
Washington, DC

Kelly Ort
GRECC, Baltimore VAMC
Baltimore, MD

Delila Parham
USDA/FSIS
Washington, DC

Mickey Parish
University of Maryland
College Park, MD

Robin E. Parsell
IOM
Washington, DC

Jill Patterson
Penn State University
University Park, PA

Nora Pihkala
USDA/FSIS/OPHS
Washington, DC

Mary Poos
FDA/Office of Nutrition, Labeling, Dietary Supplements
College Park, MD

Regis Pouillot
FDA/CFSAN
College Park, MD

Resha Putzrath
EPA
Washington, DC

P. Isaac Rabbani
FDA
College Park, MD

Rama Rachakonda
Independent Consultant
Glennn Dale, MD

Kathleen Raffaele
EPA
Washington, DC

Elizabeth Rahavi
IFIC
Washington, DC

Karen Regan
NIH
Bethesda, MD

Juliana Ruzante
University of Maryland
College Park, MD

Leila Saldanha
Company Principal
NutrIQ LLC

Morton Satin
Salt Institute
Rockville, MD

Stephanie Saullo
ADA
Washington, DC

David Schmidt
IFIC
Washington, DC

Andrew Shao
Council for Responsible Nutrition
Washington, DC

Judy R Simon
Maryland Department on Aging
Baltimore, MD

Caroline Smith DeWaal
CSPI
Washington, DC

Kathleen Smith
Smith & Associates

Thomas Sobotka
FDA/CFSAN
Silver Spring, MD

Goody Solomon
FNH News Service

Christine Spain
President's Council on Physical Fitness & Sports
Washington, DC

Barbara Spates
Genesis HealthCare
Sicklerville, NJ

Pamela Starke-Reed
NIH/DNRC
Bethesda, MD

Robert Steele
Penn State University
University Park, PA

Robin Suda
University of Maryland
College Park, MD

Ben Tall
FDA
Laurel, MD

Katherine Tallmadge
Personalized Nutrition
Washington, DC

Jennifer Teters
ADA
Washington, DC

Felicia Thompson
USDA/FSIS
Beltsville, MD

Babgaleh Timbo
FDA
College Park, MD

Rachel Tobin
SNAP-Ed Connection/FNIC/NAL/ARS
Beltsville, MD

Jane Van Doren
FDA
College Park, MD

Isabel Walls
USDA
Washighton, DC

Richetta Webb
DC Dept of Health
Washington, DC

Paddy Wiesenfeld
FDA/CFSAN
Laurel, MD

Caren Wilcox
Caren Wilcox & Associates LLC
Washington, DC

Barbara Winters
Campbell Soup Company
Camden, NJ

Donna Wixted
Genesis HealthCare
Kennett Square, PA

Derek Yach
Pepsico
Purchase, New York

Al Yamada
Masaoka & Associates, Inc.
Washington, DC

Hongyan Yang
NIH
Bethesda, MD

Melanie Young
EPA
Washington, DC

Diana Zuckerman
National Research Center for Women & Families
Washington, DC

C

Speaker, Moderator, and Panelist Biographies

Stephen Barnes, Ph.D., is a Professor in the Departments of Biochemistry and Molecular Genetics, Environmental Health Sciences, Genetics, Pharmacology and Toxicology, and Vision Sciences at the University of Alabama at Birmingham. He also serves as the Director of the Center for Nutrient-Gene Interaction, as Associate Director of the Purdue-UAB Botanicals Center for Age-Related Disease, and as Co-Director of the Comprehensive Cancer Center Mass Spectrometry/Proteomics Core Facility. His research interests include functional components of foods, and he is internationally recognized for his research on soy.

Steven Bodhaine, M.B.A., is President of the Quantitative Research Group and Director of the Global Health Practice at The Futures Company, a research-based trends and marketing consulting firm. He has counseled clients on the marketing impact of key social trends in America for the past 20 years. Mr. Bodhaine has conducted substantial primary research in the areas of new product development, branding and positioning, and marketing and communications strategy. He has focused primary attention on consulting with clients in the healthcare industry and has conducted qualitative and quantitative research among healthcare professionals, patients, policy makers, payers and the general public. Much of his work has explored the rational and emotional drivers of healthcare decision-making.

Aaron Brody, Ph.D., is President of Packaging/Brody, Inc. He is also an Adjunct Professor at the University of Georgia's Department of Food Science and Technology and teaches marketing management and new product development for M.B.A. programs at Keller Graduate School of Management and St. Joseph's University. He is an expert on the safest and best ways to package food. Dr. Brody has more than four decades of experience in food science. Working with a number of companies, he has developed precooked frozen foods, microwave food heating, modified atmosphere food preservation, aseptic packaging of high acid foods, and low-dose food irradiation.

Ronni Chernoff, Ph.D., R.D., F.A.D.A., C.S.D., is the Director of the Arkansas Geriatric Education Center, Associate Director of the Geriatric Research, Education & Clinical Center for Education and Evaluation for the Central Arkansas Veterans Affairs Health System, and Professor of Geriatrics at the University of Arkansas for Medical Sciences. She is past president of the American Dietetic Association, where she also served on the Board of Editors of the *Journal of the American Dietetic Association.* Dr. Chernoff has published numerous abstracts, journal articles, and book chapters and is editor of the text, *Geriatric Nutrition: The Health Professional's Handbook, Third Edition* (2006). She has served as Editor-in-Chief of *Perspectives in Applied Nutrition*, editor of *The Digest*, on the Editorial Board of the *Journal of Parenteral and Enteral Nutrition*, and Associate Editor of *Nutrition in Clinical Practice*. She also served on the editorial boards of *Topics in Geriatric Rehabilitation*, Nutrition Support Services, Clinical Management Newsletter, Directions in Clinical Nutrition, Senior Patient (Postgraduate Medicine), and the *Journal of Nutrition for the Elderly*. Her primary research interests are nutrition and aging and health promotion. Dr. Chernoff received her Ph.D. from the University of Pennsylvania.

Susan J. Crockett, Ph.D., R.D., F.A.D.A., is Vice President and Senior Technology Officer in Health and Nutrition at General Mills where she leads the Bell Institute of Health and Nutrition. Since 1999, she has been responsible for health and nutrition strategy and programs for General Mills' businesses, health and nutrition regulatory affairs and issues management, and nutrition science and research including dietary intake research and health professional communication.

Kerry Dearfield, Ph.D., is currently the Scientific Advisor for Risk Assessment in the U.S. Department of Agriculture's Food Safety and Inspection Service (USDA/FSIS). In the Office of Public Health Science, he develops policies, guidance, and directions for risk assessments and advises on environmental and microbial risk assessments for food safety. His scientific interests include the development of science policy and guidance; health risk assessments of environmental and microbial food contaminants; modes of action for toxicity (including mutational, physiological, and pharmacological mechanisms); use of genotoxicity data in regulatory decisions (heritable risk, carcinogenicity, general toxicity); health effects testing guidelines (e.g., carcinogenicity, mutagenicity); development and use of peer review; and, risk assessment, risk management, and risk communication issues. Prior to joining USDA, Dr. Dearfield worked as a risk assessor and Senior Scientist for Science Policy at the Environmental Protection Agency.

Caroline Smith DeWaal, J.D., is Director of Food Safety for the Center for Science in the Public Interest (CSPI). She represents CSPI in the media, in Congress, and in the regulatory arena on a broad range of food safety issues. Ms. DeWaal is CSPI's leading consumer analyst on reform of laws and regulations governing food safety. Since 1999, she has maintained and annually published a listing of foodborne illness outbreaks organized by food source that now contains over fifteen years of outbreaks reports. She has presented CSPI's outbreak database at numerous scientific conferences. She has participated in a number of World Health Organization consultations on food safety and is currently an expert advisor on its Integrated Surveillance of Antibiotic Resistance project. She represents the International Association of Consumer Food Organizations at the Codex Committee on Food Hygiene, and has participated in several national advisory committees to USDA and the Food and Drug Administration (FDA).

Michael Doyle, Ph.D., is Regents Professor of Food Microbiology and Director of the Center for Food Safety at the University of Georgia. He is an active researcher in the area of food safety and security and works closely with the food industry, government agencies, and consumer groups on issues related to the microbiological safety of foods. His research focuses on developing methods to detect and control foodborne bacterial pathogens at all levels of the food continuum, from the farm to the table. He is internationally acknowledged as a leading authority on foodborne pathogens and is a member of the Institute of Medicine.

Johanna Dwyer, D.Sc., is Senior Nutrition Scientist at the Office of Dietary Supplements (ODS) where she works under the Interagency Personnel Acquisition Program (IPA). She is also a Professor of Medicine (Nutrition) and Community Health at the Freidman School of Nutrition Science and Policy and the Tufts University Medical School, and Director of the Frances Stern Nutrition Center at Tufts-New England Medical Center. At ODS, her work involves the development of a Dietary Supplement Ingredient Database that will provide analytically substantiated values for key ingredients in dietary supplements. Dr. Dwyer also directs activities on developing understanding of dietary supplement motivation and use on the part of Americans. She is a past President of the American Society for Nutrition Sciences and the

American Society for Nutrition Education, and is a member of the National Academy of Sciences and the Institute of Medicine.

Luigi Fontana, M.D., is Research Associate Professor of Medicine at Washington University in St. Louis, as well as Associate Director of the Longevity Research Program at Washington University Medical School. He is also Director of the Division of Nutrition and Aging at the Italian National Institute of Health in Rome. Dr. Fontana has an interest in nutrition, aging, and longevity. His research focuses on the potential role of diet and exercise in retarding the aging process. Dr. Fontana is investigating the effects of calorie restriction, plant-based diets, and endurance exercise on outcomes such as cardiovascular risk factors and function, inflammation, immune function, glucose tolerance, bone metabolism, and quality of life. He is also studying the endocrine role of abdominal fat storage as a mediator of insulin resistance and accelerated aging.

Steven Gendel, Ph.D., has worked for FDA since 1990, initially at the National Center for Food Safety and Technology in Chicago as Chief of the Biotechnology Studies Branch, then with the Office of Science, and now with the Center for Food Safety and Applied Nutrition (CFSAN) Risk Assessment Coordination Team. Dr. Gendel has published extensively on the application of molecular techniques and bioinformatics to food safety and has expertise in food safety risk analysis and food safety informatics. Prior to joining FDA, he held postdoctoral positions at Harvard University and the University of Toronto and was a faculty member of the Department of Genetics at Iowa State University.

David J. Greenblatt, M.D., is Professor and Chairman of the Department of Pharmacology and Experimental Therapeutics, and Professor of Psychiatry, Medicine, and Anesthesia at Tufts University School of Medicine. He is also Director of the Clinical Pharmacology Program at Tufts University School of Medicine and Tufts Medical Center, and Associate Program Director of the institution's Clinical Research Center. Dr. Greenblatt has been an active investigator in a number of areas, including the pharmacokinetics, pharmacodynamics, and neuroreceptor properties of the benzodiazepine derivatives; drug disposition and response in old age; molecular mechanisms and consequences of drug interactions; modulation of drug metabolism by nutrients and natural medicines; and the regulation of expression and function of Cytochrome P450 enzymes and energy-dependent transport proteins. Dr. Greenblatt is also a past President of the American College of Clinical Pharmacology.

Edward Groth III, Ph.D., is a Consultant with Groth Consulting Services. His main areas of interest are food safety, toxic chemicals, risk assessment, and risk communication. He has participated, as a consumer advocate, in public debates and dialogues with government agencies on a myriad of health and safety issues.

William K. Hallman, Ph.D., is Director of the Food Policy Institute and Professor in the Department of Human Ecology at Rutgers, the State University of New Jersey. He is a psychologist with more than 20 years experience examining controversial issues related to public perceptions of risk related to food, health, and the environment. His current research projects include studies of public responses to food biosecurity threats, the use of nanotechnology in food products, and public understanding of qualified health claims.

Gordon Jensen, M.D., Ph.D., is Professor and Director of the Department of Nutritional Sciences at the Pennsylvania State University. He also serves as Professor of Medicine at the Penn State Hershey Medical Center and is a Specialist in Nutrition with Centre Medical and Surgical Associates at the Mt. Nittany Medical Center. Dr. Jensen's research interests have focused largely on geriatric nutrition concerns. He is a past President of the American Society for Parenteral and Enteral Nutrition, and past Chair of the Medical Nutrition Council of the American Society for Nutrition. Currently, Dr. Jensen is a member of the Institute of Medicine's Food and Nutrition Board and the Food Forum.

Kevin Kinsella, Ph.D., is Health Scientist Administrator and Demographer at the National Institute on Aging, Division of Behavioral and Social Research (BSR). He is responsible for the management and development of an increasingly interdisciplinary portfolio on the demography of aging. Prior to coming to BSR, he was at the U.S. Census Bureau where he served as Chief of the Aging Studies Branch in the International Programs Center, and he also served as the Study Director for two National Research Council studies. He has authored numerous publications on aging populations and prepared international demographic estimates of aging populations.

Jim Kirkwood, M.B.A., is currently Vice President of the Center for General Mills Technology Creation (G-Tech). In this role, he has leadership for a consolidated technology organization that includes the General Mills Strategic Technology Development, the Bell Institute of Health and Nutrition, GMI Materials Technology Development, GMI Agricultural Research and the company's Grain Science/Flour and Milling Technology groups. Jim brings 29 years of cross-functional experience in the food industry including assignments in research and development, marketing, general management, operations, and quality.

Jean Lloyd, M.S., has served as the National Nutritionist for the U.S. Administration on Aging in Washington, DC, since 1992. The U.S. Administration on Aging, within the Department of Health and Human Services, administers the Older Americans Act (OAA), which establishes a comprehensive and coordinated system of community-based supportive and nutrition services to older people, including congregate and home-delivered nutrition services programs. During her time with the agency, she has been responsible and provided input for the nutrition related functions of policy, budget, legislation, and regulation; program development and implementation; training and technical assistance; advocacy; evaluation; and research, demonstration, and training grants. She also represents the agency as a member of the Dietary Reference Intake Steering Committee.

Bernadene Magnuson, Ph.D., is Senior Scientific and Regulatory Consultant with Cantox Health Science and is Associate Adjunct Professor of Nutritional Sciences at the University of Toronto. Her work has focused on toxicological safety assessments of foods, dietary ingredients, and supplements, with a specific focus on cancer development. She is a pioneer in the developing field of food nanoscience, and is leading efforts to address safety issues facing the food industry in the adoption of promising new technology. Dr. Magnuson has also held multiple positions in the Institute of Food Technologists and the Society of Toxicology.

Simin Nikbin Meydani, D.V.M., Ph.D., is Director of the Jean Mayer USDA Human Nutrition Research Center on Aging at Tufts University as well as Director of the Nutritional Immunology Laboratory at the Center. She is Professor of Nutrition and Immunology at the Friedman School of Nutrition Science and Policy and Tufts Sackler Graduate Program in Immunology. Dr. Meydani's scientific interests include the impact of nutrition on immune response and resistance to infectious diseases in developed and developing countries, micronutrients, dietary lipids, calorie restriction, and probiotics, on which she has published extensively. In addition, she has studied the basic biology of aging as it is related to immune and inflammatory responses, the role of nutrition in the aging process, and age-associated diseases. Dr. Meydani has served as a member of FAO/WHO Expert Panels on nutrition and is a past President of the American Aging Association.

Marcia Pelchat, Ph.D., is Associate Member at the Monell Chemical Senses Center, an independent nonprofit institute for basic research on the chemical senses and nutrition in Philadelphia. Her major research interest is the development and modification of food and beverage preferences in humans. She is a National Institutes of Health grant reviewer, is on the editorial board of the journal, *Appetite,* and is Honorary Professor of Gastronomy at the Restaurant School in Philadelphia.

Pamela Starke-Reed, Ph.D., is Deputy Director of the National Institutes of Health's (NIH's) Division of Nutrition Research Coordination (DNRC). The DNRC advises the NIH Director and others on nutrition research issues and works with the NIH organizational components to coordinate nutrition research and research training initiatives. Prior to this position, Dr. Starke-Reed held two positions within the National Institute on Aging. Dr. Starke-Reed also serves on many committees including the Federal Steering Committee on Physical Activity Guidelines for Americans, the Federal Dietary Reference Intakes Steering Committee, and the Federal Steering Committee on Dietary Guidelines for Americans, and Healthy People 2010/2020.

Dennis Sullivan, M.D., is Director of Little Rock Geriatric Research Education and Clinical Center, Executive Vice Chairman of the Donald W. Reynolds Department of Geriatrics, and Professor of Geriatrics at the University of Arkansas for Medical Sciences. His clinical and research expertise is in the area of nutrition and rehabilitation of the frail elderly and assessment of health outcomes.

Stephen Sundlof, Ph.D., is Director of the Center for Food Safety and Applied Nutrition, Food and Drug Administration (FDA). In this capacity, he provides executive leadership to the Center's development and implementation of programs and policies relative to the composition, quality, safety, and labeling of foods, food and color additives, dietary supplements and cosmetics. Dr. Sundlof previously served as director of FDA's Center for Veterinary Medicine. Prior to joining the FDA, he was a Professor at the University of Florida, College of Veterinary Medicine.

Katherine L. Tucker, Ph.D., is Senior Scientist and Director of the Dietary Assessment and Epidemiology Research Program at the Jean Mayer USDA Human Nutrition Research Center on Aging at Tufts University. She is also Professor and Director, Nutrition Epidemiology Program for the Gerald J. and Dorothy R. Friedman School of Nutrition Science and Policy at Tufts University, and Adjunct Associate Professor for the Department of Family Medicine and Community Health at Tufts University School of Medicine. Her research interests include diet and health, nutrition in older adults, dietary methodology, nutritional status of high-risk populations, and nutrition epidemiology.

Nancy Wellman, Ph.D., is an affiliated faculty member at Tufts University's Friedman School of Nutrition Science and Policy. She recently retired as Professor of Dietetics and Nutrition in the School of Public Health at Florida International University, the public research university in Miami. She is the former director of the National Resource Center on Nutrition, Physical Activity and Aging. Dr. Wellman is a past President of the American Dietetic Association and has been a member of committees for the National Academy of Sciences and the Institute of Medicine. She currently serves as Chair of the Board of Directors for the International Food Information Council Foundation, is a member of the American Society for Nutrition (ASN) Public Information Committee, and is an ASN national spokesperson.

D

Abbreviations and Acronyms

AA	arachidonic acid (omega-6 fatty acid)
ADA	American Dietetic Association
ADME	absorption, distribution, metabolism, and excretion
AI	Adequate Intake
ASN	American Society for Nutrition
BMI	body mass index
BPA	bisphenol A
CALERIE	Comprehensive Assessment of Long-Term Effects of Reducing Intake of Energy
CDC	Centers for Disease Control and Prevention
CFSAN	Center for Food Safety and Applied Nutrition (FDA)
CPI	consumer price index
CR	caloric restriction
CSPI	Center for Science in the Public Interest
CVB3	coxsackie B3 virus
CYP3A	cytochrome P450-3A
DDT	dichlorodiphenyltrichloroethane
DHA	docosahexaenoic acid (omega-3 fatty acid)
DNRC	Division of Nutrition Research Coordination (NIH)
DRI	Dietary Reference Intake
DSHEA	Dietary Supplement Health and Education Act
DTH	delayed-type hypersensitivity

EAR	Estimated Average Requirement
EPA	eicosapentaenoic acid (omega-3 fatty acid)
FDA	Food and Drug Administration
FDC	Food, Drug, and Cosmetic Act of 1938
Fight BAC!	Fight Foodborne Bacteria
FPI	Food Policy Institute (Rutgers University)
FSIS	Food Safety and Inspection Service (USDA)
GI	gastrointestinal
GMA	Grocery Manufacturers Association
GRAS	Generally Recognized as Safe
HHS	U.S. Department of Health and Human Services
HNRCA	Jean Mayer USDA Human Nutrition Research Center on Aging (Tufts University)
IFIC	International Food Information Council
IFN-g	Interferon-gamma
IGF-1	insulin-like growth factor-1
IOM	Institute of Medicine
IU	International Unit
KO	knock-out [mice]
LDL	low-density lipoprotein
LTC	long-term care
MPa	Megapascal
NCHS	National Center for Health Statistics (CDC)
NHANES	National Health and Nutrition Examination Survey
NIA	National Institute on Aging
NIH	National Institutes of Health
NLEA	Nutrition Labeling and Education Act of 1990
NOAEL	no-observable-adverse-effect level
NORC	naturally occurring retirement community
NSAID	non-steroidal anti-inflammatory drugs
NZFSA	New Zealand Food Safety Authority
OAA	Older Americans Act
ODS	Office of Dietary Supplements (NIH)
PCA	Peanut Corporation of America

PCBs	polychlorinated biphenyls
PEEK	polyether ether ketone
PGE_2	prostaglandin E_2
psi	pounds per square inch
RDA	Recommended Dietary Allowance
RDI	Reference Daily Intake
SDS	sodium dodecyl sulfate
Se	selenium
SNAP	Supplemental Nutrition Assistance Program (USDA)
SNE	Society for Nutrition Education
STEC	Shiga toxin-producing *Escherichia coli*
S.T.O.P.	Safe Tables Our Priority
TNF	tumor necrosis factor
UK	United Kingdom
USDA	U.S. Department of Agriculture
UV	ultraviolet [light]
WIC	Supplemental Nutrition Program for Women, Infants, and Children (USDA)